WITH WORDS AND KNIVES

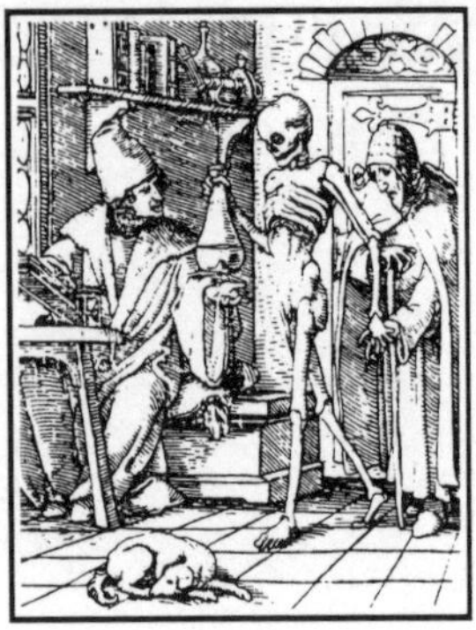

The History of Medicine in Context

Series Editors: Andrew Cunningham and Ole Peter Grell

Department of History and Philosophy of Science
University of Cambridge

Department of History
Open University

Titles in this series include:

Medicine and Religion in Enlightenment Europe
Edited by Ole Peter Grell and Andrew Cunningham

The Making of Addiction
The 'Use and Abuse' of Opium in Nineteenth-Century Britain
Louise Foxcroft

Melancholy and the Care of the Soul
Religion, Moral Philosophy and Madness in Early Modern England
Jeremy Schmidt

Hospital Politics in Seventeenth-Century France
The Crown, Urban Elites and the Poor
Tim McHugh

The Great Nation in Decline
Sex, Modernity and Health Crises in Revolutionary France c.*1750–1850*
Sean M. Quinlan

With Words and Knives

Learning Medical Dispassion in Early Modern England

LYNDA PAYNE

ASHGATE

Published by
Ashgate Publishing Limited
Gower House
Croft Road
Aldershot
Hampshire GU11 3HR
England

Ashgate Publishing Company
Suite 420
101 Cherry Street
Burlington, VT 05401-4405
USA

Ashgate website: http://www.ashgate.com

British Library Cataloguing in Publication Data
Payne, Lynda
With Words and Knives: Learning Medical Dispassion in Early Modern England. – (The History of Medicine in Context)
1. Physicians – Psychology. 2. Surgeons – Psychology. 3. Physician and patient – England – History – 16th century. 4. Physician and patient – England – History – 17th century. 5. Medicine – Practice – England – History – 16th century. 6. Medicine – Practice – England – History – 17th century. 7. Surgery – Practice – England – History – 16th century. 8. Surgery – Practice – England – History – 17th century.
I. Title
610.6’95’0942’0903

Library of Congress Cataloging-in-Publication Data
Payne, Lynda Ellen Stephenson.
With Words and Knives: Learning Medical Dispassion in Early Modern England / by Lynda Payne.
p. cm. – (The History of Medicine in Context)
Includes index.
1. Physicians – Attitudes – England – History – 17th century. 2. Physicians – Attitudes – England – History – 18th century. 3. Physician and patient – England – History – 17th century. 4. Physician and patient – England – History – 18th century. 5. Medicine – England – History – 17th century. 6. Medicine – England – History – 18th century.
I. Title. II. Series.
[DNLM: 1. Physician-Patient Relations – England. 2. Surgery – history – England. 3. History of Medicine – England. 4. History, 17th Century – England. 5. History, 18th Century – England. WO 11 FE5 P346 2007]
R487.P39 2007
610.942–dc22 2006036033

ISBN 978-0-7546-3689-2

Printed and bound in Great Britain by MPG Books Ltd, Bodmin, Cornwall.

Contents

List of Illustrations

Acknowledgments

As this book originated with my 1997 thesis, I wish to first thank the late Betty Jo Teeter Dobbs for encouraging me to pursue this topic. Her untimely death is still mourned. I am grateful to Paula Findlen for guiding me through the arduous process of writing a dissertation and to Cathy Kudlick and Hal Cook for being on my committee. I also owe a great deal to many colleagues and friends. They include Katherine Bell, Tracy Miller, Bruce Janacek, Antonio Barrera, Loretta Reed, Ellen Koehler, Jennifer D. Selwyn, Karen Halttunen, Deborah Harkness, Michael Dietrich, Joan Cadden, Karl Jacoby, E. Leigh Gibson, Sally Bragg, the late Roy Porter, Ruth Richardson, Diana Manuel, Beth Dolan, Judith Killen, David K. Robinson, Gerhild Williams and Robert Martensen.

Nearer home I am especially grateful to my colleagues in the History Department at the University of Missouri-Kansas City for their unstinting support as I weathered several personal storms. I am honoured to be associated with such gifted teachers and scholars. Members of the Faculty Interdisciplinary Workshops at UMKC gave thoughtful comments on several of the chapters. In particular I would like to thank Linda Voigts, Patricia Brodsky and Andrew Bergerson. My home away from home has been the History and Philosophy of Medicine Department at Kansas University Medical Center. In particular I would like to thank Christopher Crenner, Dawn McInnis and Frederick and Grace Holmes for stimulating discussions on many topics. In medical history classes at Oberlin College and at UMKC, undergraduates helped me think more clearly about humanity and inhumanity, passion and dispassion. Conversations with my graduate students, especially Ryan Fagan, both strengthened and problematized my thesis.

I am indebted to the librarians at the Wellcome Library, The Huntington Library, the College of Physicians of Philadelphia, the New York Academy of Medicine, the Royal College of Surgeons of London, Edinburgh University Library, the Miller Nichols Library and the Health Sciences Library at UMKC, especially Susan Sykes-Berry. I have been fortunate to receive grants and fellowships towards the research and writing of this book. I thank the New York Academy of Medicine, the Wood Institute at the College of Physicians of Philadelphia, the University of Missouri Board of Trustees, the National Endowment for the Humanities, the Woodrow Wilson Foundation, The Huntington Library, Oberlin College, the Wellcome Trust, and the University of California at Davis for all their support.

I also wish to acknowledge my medical team who helped me to cope with the diagnosis, and then get through the treatment, for advanced breast cancer. The fact that I am here today is largely due to the *passionate* care of Drs John May, Maureen Sheehan, David Robinson, Robin Hart, John Shook, Sheryl Young and, in particular, their dedicated nurses, technicians and administrative staffs. Bentley the dog also provided much needed solace during this difficult time.

I could not have had a better reader and editor than Andrew Cunningham. His consistent support and encouragement as I limped towards the final draft of the manuscript meant more than words can say.

Finally, I wish to thank my family for putting up with my fascination for the grosser aspects of medicine over many years. I dedicate this book to my dear husband Bill and to the memories of my late sister and father.

For Bill and
in memory of my little sister Sharon, 1957–2004,
and my beloved father Basil Henry Payne, 1928–2005

Introduction

In practice, physicians, and especially surgeons, have always had to learn some type of detachment (or dispassion to use the early modern term) in order to cope with the more revolting aspects of their art.[1] At times the relationship between acquiring dispassion and the effects it has on the (in)humanity of medical practitioners has been questioned. Does constantly seeing sickness and death make one lose compassion? If so, what is one left with in its place? As recently as 1994, tempers flared in the *British Medical Journal* following the publication of a letter from an anonymous London-based general practitioner. She, or he, accused some doctors of 'disturbingly callous and rude behaviour' towards patients and suggested that 'courses to remind (or perhaps teach) doctors how to behave to their patients be put high on the agenda.'[2] The letter prompted a strongly worded editorial in the *British Medical Journal* by D. J. Weatherall titled 'The inhumanity of medicine.'[3] Weatherall agreed with the sentiments of the letter and offered explanations for why so many medical practitioners appeared to be detached from their patients' pain and suffering. First, he suggested that 'doctors may always have had a limited facility to treat their patients as humans'; second, they are worse at it now 'because of the rushed and specialized nature' of medical training and practice; and third, we could try to reform medical education but there is probably little point, as 'problems of doctor-patient relationships have been around for hundreds of years and during times of completely different patterns of medical education, clinical practice, and social pressure'.[4] Weatherall ended his editorial with a plaintive cry:

> It is difficult to equate the delightful, caring, and extremely gifted young people whom one encounters on their entry to medical school with some of the horror stories described in today's journal. What on earth has exposure to a few years of the medical profession done to some of them?[5]

This book is about what exposure to medicine, especially anatomy and surgery, did to some men in early modern England.

That medical dispassion, or to use the modern term that some historians have given it, clinical detachment, has existed throughout the history of medicine is not

1 One of the best contemporary descriptions of how the practice of medicine affects one's humanity over time, is in Kaplan, Jonathan (2001), *The Dressing Station: A Surgeon's Chronicle of War and Medicine,* London: Grove Press.

2 Quoted in the editorial by D.J. Weatherall (24–31 December 1994), *British Medical Journal*, 309, p. 1672.

3 Ibid., p. 1671.

4 Ibid., p. 1672. The editorial drew a flood of letters on suggestions for humanizing medicine, from general practitioners, surgeons, pathologists and medical students.

5 *Idem.*

in question.[6] In her exhaustive study of hospital medicine, *Charitable Knowledge: Hospital Pupils and Practitioners in Eighteenth-Century London*, Susan Lawrence states that such 'attitudes were as old as systematic medical practice itself'.[7] Her analysis of Georgian ward-walking shows that this practice reinforced 'the double vision' of seeing patients as subjects and objects which is 'crucial for a practitioner's bedside authority'.[8]

In *Death, Dissection and the Destitute*, Ruth Richardson discusses how the values underlying anatomical entrepreneurship in eighteenth- and early nineteenth-century Britain transmuted the corpse from an object of veneration into a commodity to be bought and sold for scientific purposes. She mentions what effect cutting on the dead may have had on the character of early modern medical men. Richardson cites William Harvey's ability to dissect family members and William Hunter's direction to his pupils that anatomizing would familiarize their hearts to a 'necessary Inhumanity' as examples of early clinical detachment.[9]

Jonathan Sawday disagrees that anatomists sought or taught clinical detachment in the early modern era. In *The Body Emblazoned: Dissection and the Human Body in Renaissance Culture*, he sees scientific disinterest as the key to understanding dissection from the late eighteenth century onward. Before that, anatomists strove to place the body 'within a nexus of complementary discourses, so that its full symbolic significance would be appreciated by those gathered to watch its progressive disintegration'.[10] Like executioners, medical men became inured to the spectacle of suffering because it was expected of them.

In *Knowledge and Practice in English Medicine, 1550–1680*, Andrew Wear cogently argues that surgeons could not, and did not, ignore pain. Instead it was something they observed and tried to mitigate both before and during surgery. Pain was constantly being negotiated – it could lead to an operation being demanded or stop an operation from taking place.[11] Peter Stanley, in *For Fear of Pain: British Surgery, 1790–1850*, focuses on what took place at a social level in the operating room during the last decades before the development of anaesthesia. He ably

6 On the passions see Paster, Gail Kern, Rowe, Katherine, Floyd-Wilson, Mary (eds) (2004), *Reading the Early Modern Passions: Essays in the Cultural History of Emotion*, Philadelphia: University of Pennsylvania Press.

7 Lawrence, Susan (1995), *Charitable Knowledge: Hospital Pupils and Practitioners in Eighteenth-Century London,* Cambridge and New York: Cambridge University Press, p. 27.

8 Ibid., p. 340.

9 Richardson, Ruth (2001), *Death, Dissection and the Destitute*, Chicago: University of Chicago Press, p. 30. She regards Harvey's level of clinical detachment as perhaps untypical of his time period.

10 Sawday, Jonathan (1995), *The Body Emblazoned: Dissection and the Human Body in Renaissance Culture*, London and New York: Routledge, p. 63.

11 Wear, Andrew (2000), *Knowledge and Practice in English Medicine, 1550–1680*, Cambridge and New York: Cambridge University Press, p. 248.

demonstrates that, far from being hardened brutes, many surgeons feared inflicting pain and trembled, sweated and became nauseous before operating.[12]

Without a doubt early modern surgeons were aware that cutting on patients took courage, skill, and a willingness to inflict and witness great pain. Frequently texts counselled young surgeons to follow the advice of the first-century Roman encyclopaedist Celsus:

> A surgeon should be filled with pity, so that he wishes to cure his patient, yet is not moved by his cries to go too fast, or cut less than is necessary; but he does everything just as if the cries of pain cause him no emotion.[13]

A small part of Celsus' writings were transcribed and Christianized in the mediaeval surgical texts of Henri de Mondeville (1260–1320) and Guy de Chauliac (*c.*1298–1368). However, by tradition it was not until Thomas Linacre discovered a copy of all eight books of Celsus' *De re medicina* in the Archbishop of Bologna's Library that the complete works became known. They were published in 1478 and proved to be popular. The learned physician John Caius (1510–73) referred to Celsus as the 'Latin Hippocrates' and while Reader of Anatomy to the London Company of Barber-Surgeons may have popularised Celsus' writings.[14] Certainly, leading surgeons of the Company liberally quoted Celsus as the primary guide to the qualities a surgeon must exhibit to be able to operate.

In 1563 the London surgeon Thomas Gale published *An Institution of a Chirurgian conteyning the sure Groundes and Principles of Chirurgiry moste necessary and mete for those that will attayne the arte perfectly*. In it he drew on the wisdom of the ancients:

> The maners whyche GUIDO [Guy de Chauliac] woulde haue in a Chirurgian are reconed of HIPPOCRATES and CELSUS, whiche briefelye I wyll numbre; they muste be bolde and wythout feare in suche cures as are without peryll, and whereas necessitye requireth. Also in cures that bedoutful, not to be raishe and hastie, to be gentle and courtyous towarde the sicke pacient ... be mercefull towarde the pore.[15]

---

12 Stanley, Peter (2003), *For Fear of Pain: British Surgery, 1790–1850*, Amsterdam and New York: Rodopi.

13 Celsus, Aulus Cornelius (1953), 'De re medicina: Book Seven: The Prooemium,' in *Medical Works in Facsimile*, London: Pergamum Press, p. 296. Little is known of Celsus except that he was a Roman nobleman who set himself the task of epitomising, in eight great books, all contemporary science. He rated medicine as the highest science, both human and veterinary and may have been a physician.

14 The Barber-Surgeons' Company split in 1745 and the surgeons then gathered in the Corporation of Surgeons. From 1800 they were known as the Royal College of Surgeons.

15 Gale, Thomas (1596), *An Institution of a Chirurgian conteyning the sure Groundes and Principles of Chirurgiry moste necessary and mete for those that will attayne the arte perfectly*, London, p. 36. Similar passages exist in the preface to John Halle's, (1565) *An Historiall Expostulation*, London, and in William Clowes's (1596) *Profitable and Necessarie Booke*, London.

A year earlier William Bullein vividly captured the narrow road of appropriate behaviour that Celsus and Christianity had mapped out for the ideal surgeon:

> [A Surgeon] must be clenly, nimble handed, sharpe sighted, prignant witted, bolde spirited, clenly apparailed, pitefull harted, but not womanly affeccionated: to wepe or trimble, when he seeth broken bones, or bloodie woundes, neither must he geve place to the crie of his sore paciente, for softe Chyrurgians maketh fowle sores. Of the other side, he maie not plaie he partes of a Butcher to cutte, rende, or teare, the bodies of manne kynde ... for it is the pleasure of God, to cal It his temple, his instrument, and dwelying place, and the Philosopher dooe call it *Orbiculus*, that is a little world.[16]

Celsus' works remained popular into the eighteenth century. In 1756 the physician James Grieve translated *A. Cornelius Celsus of Medicine In Eight Books* and dedicated it to his anatomy teacher, Mr. Samuel Sharp at Guy's Hospital. Grieve included Celsus' advice with its stress on dispassionate affect:

> A surgeon ought to be young, or at most middle aged, to have a strong and steddy hand ... to have a quick and clear sight; to be bold, and so far void of pity, that he may have only in view the cure of him, whom he has taken in hand, and not in compassion to his cries either make more haste that the case requires, or cut less than is necessary; but to do all, as if he was not moved by the shrieks of his patient.[17]

Celsus' admonition to remain steady and focus on the operation and not on the patient's pain was a tough assignment. This book discusses how medical practitioners wrestled with their emotions and those of their patients through an examination of training, especially in anatomy, from 1600–1800 in England. Each chapter considers an 'emotional community' of medical men. This notion is borrowed from mediaeval studies, especially the work of Barbara Rosenwein.[18] In her essay 'Worrying about Emotions in History' she calls for historians to consider and analyze the emotional communities, or systems of feelings, that individuals in any time period and culture belonged to. The expression and repression of emotions within the communities of family, guild or profession were markers of communal bonds. Such communities included those of the anatomists and the surgeons in early modern England.

As in other cultures and historical eras, the learning of dispassion was enthusiastically promoted and vehemently attacked by both medical and literary writers throughout the early modern period. To elucidate what was medical dispassion in seventeenth- and eighteenth-century England, how and why it was

---

16 Bullein, William (1562), *Bullein's Bulwarke of Defence Againste all Sicknes, Sornes, and Woundes*, London, f. viij. Bullein was a rector in Suffolk and had medical training.

17 Grieve, James (1756), *A. Cornelius Celsus of Medicine In Eight Books*, London, p. 378.

18 Rosenwein, Barbara (June 2002), 'Review Essay: Worrying about Emotions in History,' *American History Review* 107 (3), pp. 821–45. On the history of emotions see Reddy, William M. (2001), *The Navigation of Feeling: A Framework for the History of Emotions*, Cambridge and New York: Cambridge University Press, and Stearns, Peter N. and Stearns, Carol Z. (October 1985) 'Emotionology: Clarifying the History of Emotions and Emotional Standards,' *American History Review*, 90, pp. 813–36.

taught, to whom and in what spaces, each chapter of the book examines an emotional community of practitioners and explores different patterns of medical education, clinical practice, social institutions and philosophical, and religious ideas.

The first chapter analyzes the effects of systematically dismembering the dead on the attitudes and emotions of early modern medical men toward the living. I focus on the most famous anatomist in early modern Europe, William Harvey (1578–1657). As a medical student at the University of Padua, Harvey was exposed to methods of dealing with death and the destruction of the human body in the sanitized milieu of the theatre of anatomy and the chaotic wards of local hospitals. He found the dead body to be a source of enormous theoretical fascination and practical satisfaction. Harvey carried out or supervised hundreds of private dissections including those of his father and sister. The subsequent fame of his work led prominent physicians and surgeons to champion a more anatomical approach to understanding and treating the body. Harvey's stress on relying on the eyes rather than texts to reveal the truth was also crucial in constructing the image of the dissecting-medical man. In 1659, when John Finch was appointed Professor of Anatomy at Pisa, he was lauded for being the ideal Harveian anatomist, 'keen in mind, a lynx with the knife, clever with a learned tongue, you cut everything, you see everything, and you are silent about nothing'.[19] The activities of Harvey and his followers did not escape the notice of the public. Stories began to circulate regarding the bizarre nature of those who dissected for a living, and a particular stereotype emerged of a stoic but flamboyant and deeply troubling, anatomist-physician.

As anatomical skill could discipline the eyes, placing reason in control of the passions could discipline the head or mind. Changing philosophical values in the seventeenth century laid the groundwork for the emergence of a new ideal type of medical practitioner – one who was able to realize the melding of knowledge, values and experience. The second chapter examines philosophical changes, such as the rise of NeoStoicism, Epicurean and Cartesian thought, or materialist approaches to the human body and their relationship to dispassion. NeoStoicism and Epicureanism provided some ingredients for the image of a disciplined practitioner while Cartesianism allowed learned medical men to imagine the body as insensible brute matter in motion. The physician Walter Charleton was an admirer of Harvey and wrote on the nature of the passions over several decades. He devoted time to studying his own emotional responses to unhappiness and pain and adapted a classical play for the stage in London. *The Ephesian Matron* (1668) has been largely ignored by historians of science and medicine. However, the intertwining of Charleton's NeoStoic interests and anatomical knowledge with his fascination for the passions is as evident in this work as in his 'purely' medical ones.

Religious developments from the 1640s provided a new basis for accepting anatomy not simply as a medical technique but as part of a broader, moral pursuit of knowledge. The English Civil War with its sectarian radicalism forged a new religious climate in the later seventeenth century that identified 'enthusiasm' and 'atheism' as public evils. Such concerns lent religious credence to the philosophical

---

19 Malloch, Archibald (1917), *Finch and Baines: A Seventeenth Century Friendship*, Cambridge: Cambridge University Press, p. 27.

emphasis on discipline and reason that had already given anatomy a new place in public discussions of scientific knowledge. The importance of religious and philosophical changes during this period in changing the culture of anatomy, and more generally medical practice, is demonstrated in the third chapter through a close analysis of the 16-volume diary of the clergyman-anatomist John Ward (1629–81). Ward was part of the generation at Oxford that included Thomas Willis, Robert Boyle, Richard Lower, Walter Needham, Christopher Wren, John Locke, Robert Hooke and John Mayow. His diaries reveal the 'self-fashioning' of an ideal Christian anatomist. Through empirical practice came spiritual self-understanding, Christian morality and the ability to detach oneself from the suffering of self and others.

The fourth chapter focuses on surgical practice in early eighteenth-century London. In recent years the image of Georgian medical practitioners as beholden to their patients has been highlighted, with medicine being viewed as a commodity to be bought and sold. However, this analysis has been balanced by accounts of the complex negotiations that often took place between patient and doctor over the subjective process of making a diagnosis and agreeing on a treatment. Examining the career and case histories of the prolific medical writer, surgeon and physician, Dr Daniel Turner (1667–1741) shows the changing therapeutic scope and status of surgery and the increasing normalization of anatomical training as the basis of medicine. In Turner's nitty-gritty world of treating both private patients and charity hospital cases, the heady philosophizing of Walter Charleton about the passions and John Ward's invocations of Seneca might not seem to have had a role to play. However, Turner's case histories provide a microcosm of the moral stance of an early modern, licensed medical practitioner towards his patients, their illnesses, the behaviour of bedside bystanders and other healers.

The eighteenth century was a watershed for the normalization of anatomical training and the rising status of surgeons and surgery. It was also a period in which one sees the values underlying medical training and practice expressed most explicitly. The final two chapters focus on the brothers William and John Hunter, their anatomy schools, teaching techniques and the shaping of their pupils. William Hunter characterized anatomic inquiry as 'the passive submission of dead bodies' and taught that:

> It is dissection alone that can teach us, where we may cut the living body, with freedom & dispatch; and where we may venture, with great circumspection and delicacy, and where we must not, upon any account attempt it. This informs the *head*, gives dexterity to the *hand*, and familiarises the *heart* with a sort of *necessary inhumanity*, the use of cutting instruments upon our fellow-creatures.[20]

---

20 See, for example, Anonymous, (*c.*1780) *Introductory Lecture of Mr. William Hunter*, St Thomas's Hospital, MS 55, f. 182v, and *Hunter's Lectures of Anatomy* (1972), Amsterdam: Elsevier Publishing Company. The latter is a facsimile of two notebooks of 185 leaves and 114 leaves. It has a date of 1752 on f. 2 in the second notebook. The two books consist of 48 lectures taken down in some form of shorthand by Charles White of Manchester in William Hunter's course which started on 20 January 1752. They were later transcribed by White or a member of the family.

Much like Celsus, Hunter's words were later paraphrased by his pupils in their own lectures to young medical men in Britain and America. I conclude that anatomical and surgical training did not just fully educate all the senses of young medical men but was also a gift of moral forbearance and dispassion. In repeated dissections, William and John Hunter informed their students' heads and gave dexterity to their hands, and so linked an intellectual penetration of the body to an instrumental penetration. This familiarized the students' hearts to a sort of 'necessary inhumanity' when it came to treating patients, performing their autopsies or snatching their bodies.

Chapter One

Faithful Eyes

> Harvey did not trust other mens writings, but his own faithfull eys, the truest reporters of Anatomy, because Anatomy is better gain'd by ocular inspection than by long reading.[1]

> Does your skilled hand make me bold?
> It has![2]

Every culture has its rules for behaviour including training in how to express or repress feelings in certain situations. This chapter seeks to understand part of the emotional community of early modern medical practitioners in England through an analysis of the attitudes of anatomists to the human body.[3] What was the effect of anatomizing on the feelings of seventeenth-century medical men towards the bodies of the dead, the living and their own bodies? How did others in and out of the community of anatomists respond to the popularization of dissecting? How did they feel about anatomists and the claim that cutting on the dead led to more knowledgeable treatment of the living? A strong model in answering these questions is the most famous anatomist in Europe, the discoverer of the circulation of the blood, William Harvey.[4]

Harvey (1578–1657) came from a merchant family in London, attended Gonville and Caius College, Cambridge as an undergraduate and received his Medical Doctorate from the University of Padua in 1602. As a medical student at Padua, Harvey was exposed along with his peers to ideals for dealing with the pain of the living and the dismemberment of the dead in the hospital and the theatre of

---

1 *The Anatomical Exercises of Dr. William Harvey with the Preface of Zachariah Wood Physician of Roterdam* [sic] (1653), London, The Preface, p. 11. This was the first English edition. Part of this chapter appeared in Payne, Lynda (December 2002), 'With much nausea, loathing, and foetor: William Harvey, dissection and dispassion in early modern medicine.' *Vesalius: Acta Internationales Historiae Medicinae*, 3 (2), pp. 45–52.

2 Keynes, Geoffrey (1966), *The Life of William Harvey*, Oxford: Clarendon Press, p. 111. This is part of a poem by Dr Peter Browne (1575–1624) in *Pseudo-medicorum anatomia* (1624). The pamphlet included Latin verses praising the President and Fellows of the College, including Browne's on Harvey.

3 See Rosenwein, B. (3 June 2002), 'Review Essay: Worrying about Emotions in History', *American History Review*, 107, pp. 821–45.

4 For Harvey's biographical details see Keele, Kenneth D. (1965), *William Harvey: The man, the physician, and the scientist*, London and Edinburgh: Thomas Nelson Printers Ltd., Keynes, Geoffrey (1966), *The Life of William Harvey*, Oxford: Clarendon Press, French, Roger (1994), *William Harvey's Natural Philosophy*, Cambridge: Cambridge University Press.

anatomy. He apparently became quite addicted to investigating the dead. Harvey would go on to carry out and witness many private dissections including those of his father and sister. In anatomical lectures to the College of Physicians he matter-of-factly included the 'huge colon in father' and 'large spleen in my sister 5lb' as case materials to illustrate certain anomalies.[5] In 1602 Harvey set up practice in London. Two years later he became a primary physician to Saint Bartholomew's Hospital and a licentiate of the College of Physicians. Harvey was physician extraordinary to James I and physician-in-ordinary to Charles I. In 1616 he was appointed to the post of Lumleian Lecturer in Anatomy and Surgery to the College, which required him to hold a five-day dissection of a body every winter.[6] In the Lumleian lectures to the College, Harvey sought to provide his colleagues with the anatomical education he had acquired at Padua. As was becoming increasingly common in European dissections, Harvey lectured and dissected simultaneously. He occasionally identified dead patients and their diseases.[7] For example, along with his father and sister Harvey mentioned the autopsies of his cousin's husband, the Earl of Leicester's daughter, Lord Chichester and the anonymous cadavers of the sick poor at St Bartholomew's Hospital. With the President of the College of Physicians, John Argent, Harvey examined the meninges of Argent's daughter and the heart of Argent's relative, Sir Robert Darcy. This tradition of anatomy in the family and the naming of dead patients probably represented an increasing familiarity with handling bodies and a desire to advertise the use of anatomy to households and individuals. It perhaps even acted to encourage autopsies as an ordinary and desirable part of medicine, a situation Katherine Park has similarly argued for Renaissance Italy.[8]

In 1628 Harvey published *Exercitatio anatomica de motu cordis et sanguinis in animalibus* in which he told his readers that he had reached his conclusions about the circulation of the blood, 'by autopsy on the live and the dead, by reason [and] by experiment.'[9] As is well known, Harvey's observations of the circulation of the blood met with a mixed response at best. The diarist John Aubrey reported that Harvey told him, 'that after his booke of the Circulation of the Blood came-out, that he fell mightily in his practize, and that 'twas beleeved by the Vulgar that he was

5 Harvey, William (1961), *Lectures on the Whole of Anatomy: An Annotated Translation of Prelectiones Anatomiae Universalis*, O'Malley, C.D., Poynter, F.N.L. and Russell, K.F. (eds), Berkeley: University of California Press, p. 75. Kenneth Keele reported that in Harvey's published works alone he found 63 specific references to post-mortems performed by him. Keele estimated that Harvey must have dissected an additional 40–50 hanged men in the course of the Lumelian Lectures. See 'William Harvey as Morbid Anatomist', (August 1962), *Proceedings of the Royal Society of Medicine*, 55, pp. 677–85.

6 On the creation of the surgical lecture in 1581 by Richard Caldwell and Lord Lumley see Harvey, *Lectures on the Whole of Anatomy*, pp.1–11.

7 Harvey used English to describe his cases and personal recollections because Latin would have been difficult given its limited medical vocabulary, notes French in *William Harvey's Natural Philosophy*. Perhaps English was also used to entertain the less medically minded visitors at his lectures?

8 See Park, Katharine (1994), 'The Criminal and Saintly Body: Autopsy and Dissection in Renaissance Italy', *Renaissance Quarterly*, 47, pp. 1–33.

9 Harvey, *Lectures on the Whole of Anatomy*, pp.76 and 99.

crack-brained; and all the physitians were against his opinion ... .'[10] However by 1653 Harvey was being lauded in verse by Commonwealth poet Martin Lluelyn as the wielder of a knife that had made 'living laboratories of the beasts' for 'there thy Observing Eye first found the Art /Of all the Wheels and Clock-work of the Heart.'[11] The Cartesian overtones are unmistakable.

In 1654 the Harveian Museum, with its 1,280 titles in the medical sciences and natural philosophy, eight dozen dissecting and surgical instruments and an equal number of preparations, was opened to great fanfare at the College of Physicians. Two years later Harvey was elected President of the College, an honour he declined because of ill health and age.[12] His endowments were recognized with poems and speeches praising his discoveries and heroic character. Harvey needed 'not a club, but only his dissecting knife to slay the seven-headed hydra of error.'[13]

In just over 20 years Harvey had been elevated by his peers from 'crack-brained' to the founding father of English anatomy. This was as much due to his invention of a successful method of practising human dissection and animal vivisection that could be easily replicated as it was to the discovery of the circulation of the blood. In London from the late 1630s and later at Oxford during the siege between May and June 1645, Harvey accumulated admirers who, individually and then collectively, undertook research projects in anatomy. Physicians such as George Ent, Francis Glisson, Nathaniel Highmore, Thomas Wharton, Walter Charleton, William Petty and Thomas Willis investigated anatomy through repeated dissections of felons, vivisection of animals and post-mortems of private patients. They made visible and published the 'new knowledge' of which Harvey had spoken and linked it to fevers, ferments and diseases.[14]

---

10 Aubrey, John (1898), *Brief Lives,* ed. Andrew Clark, Oxford: Clarendon Press, 1, p. 300.

11 Martin Lluelyn or Llewellyn was a doctor who had been with Harvey at the Oxford siege. See Frank, Jr, Robert G. (1979), 'The Image of Harvey in Commonwealth and Restoration England', in Bylebyl, Jerome J. (ed.), *William Harvey and His Age: The Professional and Social Context of the Discovery of Circulation*, Baltimore: John Hopkins University Press, pp. 103–36, information from p. 123. Like Francis Drake, Harvey had become a '*Circulator* (but) of the *Lesser World.*' Jonathan Sawday discusses Lluelyn in *The Body Emblazoned.* Harvey's *De generatione animalium* appeared in 1653 in an English translation (Latin edition, 1651). It was prefaced with celebratory verses by Martin Lluelyn 'which set a tone that was deeply misogynist' and celebrated Harvey as the heroic male scientist 'in a language of potency', p. 238.

12 See Frank, 'The Image of Harvey', pp. 114–15.

13 Frank, Robert (1979), *English Scientific Virtuosi in the 16th and 17th Centuries*, Los Angeles: William Andrews Clark Library, p. 100, quoting Dr John Collop in 1656 before the College.

14 George Ent defended the circulation of the blood in *Apologia pro circulatione sanguinis* (1641). Francis Glisson wrote a clinical treatise on rickets *De rachitide* (1650) and on the liver *Anatomia hepatis* (1654). Nathaniel Highmore's *Corporis humani disquisitio anatomica* (1651) supported Harvey's anatomical method, while Thomas Wharton's *Adenographia* (1656) detailed new discoveries on the glands. Walter Charleton's *Oeconomia animalis* (1659) discussed physiology. Thomas Willis in *Diatribae duae* (1659) applied anatomy to fevers and ferments. See Frank, 'The Image of Harvey'. He describes a network of at least two dozen

The training of an anatomist

William Harvey may well have witnessed a dissection as a student at Gonville and Caius College, Cambridge. However the roots of Harvey's later investigations lay in the education he received in medical Galenism and the humanist tradition of anatomy while a medical student at the University of Padua from 1599 to 1602.[15] By the later sixteenth century the idea of anatomy developed by Vesalius had become firmly fixed at Italian universities. The authority of anatomy was established through a carefully managed public spectacle, pedagogical techniques whereby it was promoted as a distinct discipline within the medical tradition and a construction of the body by the lecturer as the authoritative source of knowledge. Harvey's first exposure to the systematic medical dismemberment of the human body probably occurred within the purpose-built theatre of anatomy at the University of Padua.[16] There, Harvey developed certain mechanisms of adjustment and defence during his early clinical training.[17]

The theatre was built between 1593 and 1594 in the shape of a funnel and although only 10 by 7.5 metres (33 by 25 feet) across, had room for two to three hundred standing spectators. As no daylight penetrated, it was lit by two chandeliers with four candles each and eight candles held by the students. Harvey was the head, or Chancellor, of the English nation of students at Padua and would presumably have sat in the second or third tier.[18] Conditions during the public anatomies Harvey witnessed would have been overcrowded and dark, while the smell emanating from the cadaver and the excited crowd must have been oppressive.[19]

---

anatomists working in Oxford, Cambridge and London which 'had its origin in Harvey', p. 106.

15 See Jones, Peter Murray (1988), 'Thomas Lorkyn's Dissections,1564/5 and 1566/7', in *Transactions of the Cambridge Bibliographical Society*, 9, pp. 209–29. Jones concludes, 'It is clear that in the 1560's at least dissection did take place, and was attended by men who went on to become leaders of the medical profession', p. 226. Keynes speculates that Harvey's reference to the small liver and spleen that he had seen in a corpse at Cambridge in the Lumleian lectures suggests he may have attended a dissection there, *The Life of William Harvey*, p. 11.

16 For a detailed discussion of the anatomy theatre at Padua, see Klestinec, Cynthia (2004), 'A History of Anatomy Theaters in Sixteenth-Century Padua', *Journal of the History of Medicine and Allied Sciences*, 59 (3), pp. 375–412.

17 On Harvey's time at Padua see Berti-Bock, G., Premuda, L., Vial, F., Rulliere, R., (1980) 'Le séjour de William HARVEY à Padoue', *Histoire des Sciences Medicales*, 14 (1), pp. 317–24, and Whitteridge, Gweneth (1971), *William Harvey and the Circulation of the Blood*, London: Macdonald.

18 Castiglioni, Arturo (May 1941), 'The Origin and Development of the Anatomical Theater to the End of the Renaissance', *Ciba Symposia*, 3, (2), pp. 826–44. Also see Lunsingh Scheurleer, Th. H. (1975), 'Un Amphithéâtre D'Anatomie Moralisée', in Th. H. Lunsingh Scheurleer and G.H.M. Posthumus Meyjes (eds), *Leiden University in the Seventeenth Century: An Exchange of Learning*, Leiden: Leiden University Press, pp. 217–77. The theatre at Leiden was much larger, better lit and airier than Padua.

19 See Bylebyl, Jerome (1987), 'The School of Padua: Humanistic Medicine in the Sixteenth Century,' in Charles Webster (ed.), *Health, Medicine and Mortality in the Sixteenth*

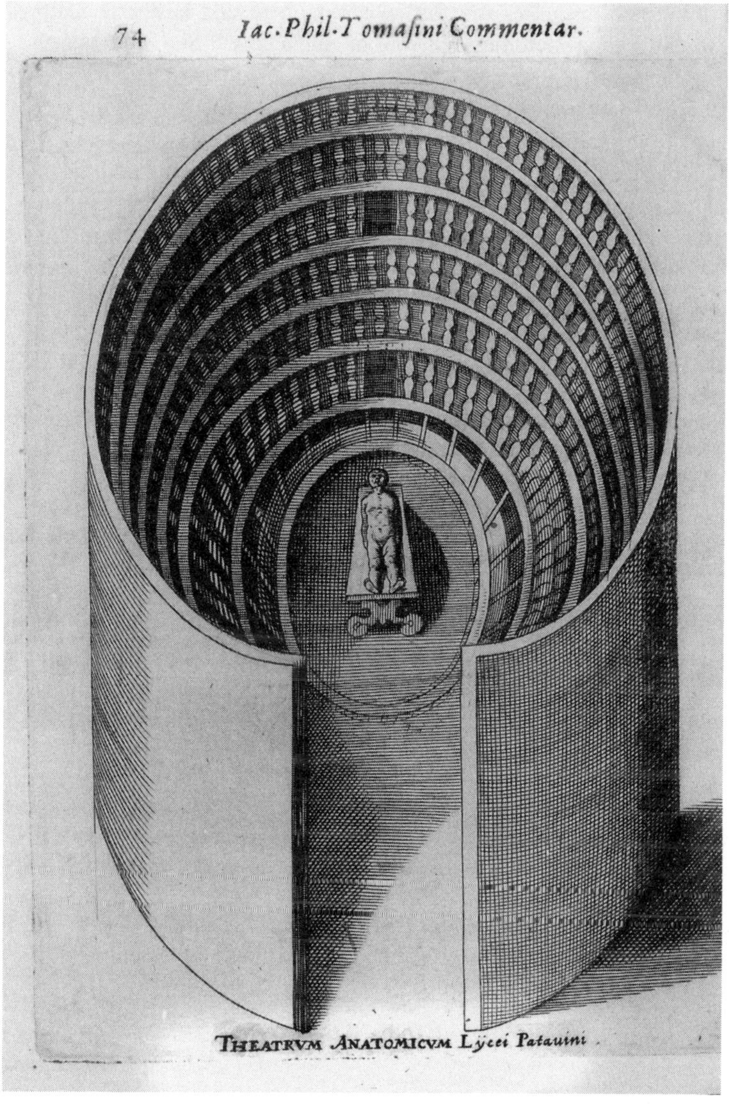

Figure 1.1 The anatomy theatre of Padua in the late sixteenth century. From G. F. Tomasini, *Gymnasium Patavinum ... Ultini*, 1654. By kind permission of the Clendening Library.

Century, Cambridge: Cambridge University Press, pp. 361–63, for more details on Padua. Also see Ferrari, Giovanna (November 1987), 'Public Anatomy Lessons and the Carnival in Bologna', *Past and Present*, 117, pp. 50–106, Rupp, Jan (1990), 'Matters of Life and Death: the social and cultural conditions of the rise of anatomical theaters, with special reference to seventeenth century Holland', *History of Science*, 28, pp. 264–87 and Rupp (March 1992), 'Michel Foucault, Body Politics and the Rise and Expansion of Modern Anatomy, *Journal of Historical Sociology*, 5 (1), pp. 31–59.

Cynthia Klestinec discusses the formal atmosphere and aesthetic features of the new theatre in Padua including the role of musicians.[20] She contrasts the style of Vesalius – constantly dissecting and talking to his students, encouraging questions and touching of the body – to that of Fabricius who focused on the exposition of the causes of human nature. Fabricius was one of Harvey's professors and appears to have encouraged his students to listen to his philosophical musings on the body rather than touch and ask questions.[21] Klestinec concludes that in the late sixteenth century two styles of anatomy evolved at Padua. One was a low style, oriented around dissection, structural anatomy and the students. It was much like the format of their private lessons and probably took place in the rooms under the main theatre floor.[22] The high style developed in public demonstrations that promoted and published the symbolic significance of anatomy.[23] In the 1590s when Harvey was a student:

> Students continued to seek private instruction, associating it with the comprehensive treatment of the body and the opportunity to see and perhaps practice surgical operations ... . In private settings, they asked questions, participating in the labors of their own intellectual development. In public settings ... they attended the university event, watched the entrance of important university officials and professors, appreciated the decor of the theater, and awaited the pleasant sounds of music and orations on the nature of man.[24]

At least when it came to public demonstrations, Continental anatomy theatres were meant to be harmonious spaces. There the body could be presented, in a pleasant fashion as the foremost example of the wisdom of God, to the audience of future physicians and interested dignitaries. Johann Vesling, Professor in Anatomy at Padua during the 1640s, stated in the preface to his volume on anatomy:

> I framed this smal [sic] Work, in the manner as we shew it in publick Dissections of the Body of Man: I avoided Controversies, which belong rather to Contemplatists, than the Theatres of Anatomists, *which were built to behold, not to dispute in.*[25]

What do we know about the role of the anatomist at public events and how the audience may have emotionally responded to listening and watching a dissection in progress?

---

20 Klestinec, p. 380.

21 Ibid., p. 381.

22 For more information on Renaissance anatomy including which bodies were chosen for dissection, see Carlino, Andrea (1999), *Books of the Body: Anatomical Ritual and Renaissance Learning*. Chicago: University of Chicago Press. This was originally published as *La Fabbrica Del Corpo: Libri e dissezione nel Rinascimento*, Torino: Giulio Einaudi editore in 1994.

23 Klestinec, p. 410.

24 Ibid., p. 403

25 Veslingus, Johannes (1653), *The Anatomy of the Body of the Man, wherein is exactly describes every part therof, in the same manner as it is commonly shewed in Publick Anatomies,* London. Johann Vesling was Chair of Anatomy at Padua and his work was translated from the Latin by Nicholas Culpeper.

A sense of the visual feast presented by anatomizing to the audience at Padua was captured in the diary of the naturalist John Evelyn. In 1646 he watched Vesling dissect and lecture:[26]

> [I] went to Padoa to be present at the famous Anatomie lecture, which is here celebrated with extraordinary apparatus, lasting almost a whole moneth. During this time I saw a woman, a child, and a man dissected with all the manual operations of chirurgeon on the humane body. The one was performed by Cavalier Vestlingius and Dr. Jo Athelsteinius Leonaenas ... When the Anatomie Lectures, which were in the mornings, were ended, I went to see cures don in the Hospitals ... .[27]

Evelyn was so impressed by the skill of the anatomists when it came to cutting on the body that he purchased a large and expensive souvenir, a 'rare Tables of Veines and Nerves, and caus'd him [Leonaenas] to prepare a third of the Lungs, Liver, and Nervi sexti par; with the Gastric Veines.'[28]

A description of anatomy at the University of Padua also comes from John Finch (1626–82). Finch was related to William Harvey, and his father Heneage Finch, witnessed Harvey's will.[29] In one of his notebooks Finch copied out a Latin poem written by his companion and fellow Padua medical student, Thomas Baines, in praise of their Professor of Anatomy, Antonio Molinetti.[30] Baines first commented upon the many 'stupendous things' we have seen in the bodies 'to which you apply your hand':[31]

---

26 Vesling and Harvey corresponded and the former's book, *Syntagma anatomicum*, with its praise of Harvey's discovery of the circulation of the blood was used as a tutorial text at Oxford in the 1650s by the head of Hart Hall, Philip Stephens. See Frank, 'The Image of Harvey', p. 112.

27 (1819) *Memoirs illustrative of the life and writings of John Evelyn ... edited by William Bray,* London, p. 203.

28 Evelyn presented the tables to the Royal Society in 1667. See *Musaeum Regalis Societatis or a catalogue and description of the natural and artificial rarities belonging to the Royal Society*, London, Printed by W. Rawlins, for the Author, 1681. 'All the Principal VEINS, ARTERIES, and NERVES, both of the Limbs and Viscera. The generous Gift of John Evelyn Esquire. He brought them at Padoa, where he saw them with great industry and exactness (according to the best method then used) taken out of the body of a Man, and very curiously spread upon four large TABLES, whereon they are now preserved.' p. 4.

29 Heneage Finch became Lord Chancellor and Earl of Nottingham.

30 In 1649 the Venetian Antonio Molinetti succeeded Vesling as Professor of Anatomy at Padua. Molinetti especially studied the sense organs. On his work see Bosatra, Andrea (1954), 'L'organo dell'udito negli studi di Antonio Molinetti anatomico padovano del '600', *Minerva otorinolaringologica,* 4, pp. 99–102.

31 Malloch, Archibald (1917), *Finch and Baines: A Seventeenth Century Friendship*, Cambridge: Cambridge University Press, p. 15. Malloch provided both the Latin and the translation. I am very grateful to Andrew Cunningham for correcting the last stanza of the poem. 'Stupenda vidimus! ... Molinette sic decet queis admoves manum ... . p.14. The poem was written in the notebook in 1662 but is probably from 1652–56 when Finch and Baines were medical students at Padua. On John Finch and his career see Villani, Stefano (2005), 'Between Anatomy and Politics: John Finch and Italy, 1649–1671' in Pelling, Margaret and

> But hear, kind Father, the gentle complainings of thy children ... you solve all enigmas and you weave knots. We cease to wonder at man; but a new labour arises: we begin to be amazed at Molinetti alone. While you search the supple pathways of the blood, its nimble course, its slippery passages, behold our own blood seized with ecstasy, halts inert in our veins ... you do not dissect bodies, Molinetti, but adorn them. You bring them into the Theatre cleansed from all dirt, perfectly in limb, and the obedient muscles are freed at your touch; thus you do not display yourself, the anatomist, but what is far greater, God.[32]

Baines's gentle satire supports Klestinec's argument that high and low styles of anatomy evolved at Padua. Here the body is presented in the high style, sanitized and at the command of a somewhat jaded anatomist who 'adorns' bodies rather than 'dissects' them.

What emotions are elicited and repressed here? First, there is awe at the abilities of Molinetti to deconstruct the body with words and knives. In fact, Molinetti is so skilled at deconstructing the body that it ceases to exist for the students; instead, the living body of the anatomist becomes the focus of the dissection. Second, there is reverence. As Molinetti reveals the dead body to be no mystery, the students 'cease to wonder' at it and instead focus on the anatomist – 'we begin to be amazed at Molinetti alone.' Third, as the students switch from watching the body to watching Molinetti, they become conscious of their own bodies – 'behold our own blood seized with ecstasy, halts inert in our veins.' Finally, there is pleasure in the beauty of the corpse, the 'them' that respond to the commands of the anatomist. As Vesling stated in the preface to *The Anatomy of the Body of the Man* the theatre can function as a contemplative space in which reverential conditions are produced and one can behold God. In this case God is worshipped through the skills of the anatomist who acts as an earthly conduit revealing the wonders of the universe to 'thy children'.

In 1659 the same John Finch was appointed Professor of Anatomy at the University of Pisa. He appears to have learned his lesson well from Molinetti for Finch was lauded at his inauguration for being the ideal anatomist – 'keen in mind, a lynx with the knife, clever with a learned tongue, you cut everything, you see everything, and you are silent about nothing.'[33] The sharpness of Finch's mind, knife and tongue represented the emotional honing his head, hands and heart had received as a student of Molinetti's.[34]

Mandelbrote, Scott (eds), *The Practice of Reform in Health, Medicine, and Science,1500–2000*, Aldershot and Burlington, VT: Ashgate, pp.151–166.

32 'Sed filiorum sentias clemens Pater/ Dulces querelas, quas vagientes proferunt/ Enigmaes omnes solvis, et nectis nodos/ Desinimus adnirari hominem, at novus labor/ Incipimus unum obstupescere Molinettum/ Qui flexusos sanguinis dum tramites/ Agilemque cursum permeatus lubricos/ Scrutaris, en sanguis correptus extasi/ Stat piger in venis, nescitque progredi/ Quia cum stupore viderat motum suum ... Dissectiones laudent queis placent tuas/ Parcius oportet istas: nam me judice/ Non dissecas Molinette sed adornas corpora/ Et sordibus remotis, in crus integrum/ Producis in Theatrum, et sequaces musculi/ Solvuntur ad tactum; sic non Te Anatomicum/ Praestas sed id quod abunde magis est, Deum.' Malloch, p.15.

33 Malloch, p. 27.

34 In 1661 Thomas Baines succeeded William Petty as Professor of Music at Gresham College. Villani, p. 156.

Dissections appear to have elicited feelings of awe, satisfaction and pleasure in students. They were excited and fascinated by the skill of the anatomist and passionate about his manipulation of the body. Such passion may have acted to repress any feelings of disgust at the sight of a dismembered body. However, living bodies were not clean, still or obedient and caused different emotions in students. When exposed to the more chaotic clinical rounds and post mortems at the Hospital of San Francesco that adjoined the University of Padua, distance from the body was far less achievable.

By the late sixteenth century, daily hospital rounds with formal discussion of major cases, systematic teaching of urines and pulses, and autopsies of fatal cases were part of the medical education at Padua. It quickly became apparent that the foreign students came to Padua because of the bedside precepting or practical training in medicine. After all, they could get the theory at home. Most foreign students, including William Harvey, had taken their first degrees where practical medicine was not available.[35] In 1597 they protested when the Moderators of the University tried to restrict visiting of the sick due to poor attendance at the public (high style) lectures. As a medical student following the great Fabricius or some other professor around the crowded wards of San Francesco Hospital, watching them first treat then dissect patients, Harvey would have been exposed to practical methods of dealing with suffering, death and the dismemberment of the human body. His memories of the hospital, along with his later experiences as the primary physician to St Bartholomew's Hospital in London, suggest that there were some situations in which even Harvey had difficulty overcoming his emotional reaction.[36]

While discussing differing types of liver abscesses, some 'Hard from tension ... like a heape of pus of pale yellow colour ... .' Harvey commented, 'I observed these things in the hospital (Saint Bartholomew's) as well as in the hospitals of Italy with much nausea, loathing, and foetor. I have forgotten many things.'[37] The use of 'forgotten' is telling as is the reaction to the liver abscesses that Harvey experienced. What disturbed him was the smell which provoked nausea and the subsequent loathing and foetor. Harvey also recognized that he had forgotten or tried to repress many olfactory memories of the patients he saw. Such a defence mechanism was vital if he was to open bodies and explore their decaying contents.

No doubt the dissection of the abdominal region presented Harvey with the prime example of the cadaver as an aesthetically repulsive object, 'Ist. lower venter, nasty yet recompensed by admirable variety ... .' he wrote in his lecture notes. As the largest cavity in the human body, fluids naturally collected there and nondescript organs such as the soft and slippery intestines would be full of undigested food and faecal matter at times. When opened, this resulted in a horrendous stench. Moreover, in the summer heat of Italy, rancid fat must have flowed through the hands of the dissector as he worked in the abdominal region.

---

35 Bylebyl, 'The School of Padua', especially pp. 350–51.

36 Bylebyl confirms that there were daily hospital rounds with formal discussion of major cases and autopsies of fatal cases in the late sixteenth century at the hospital of San Francesco, 'The School of Padua', p.364.

37 Whitteridge, p. 14.

The physician Thomas Wharton, an admirer of Harvey, performed an autopsy on a judge in the summer of 1673 in Cornwall. 'Despite the smell soe violent and offensive to us all' he opened the body 'being overborne with the curiousity of finding something of the realityes of the cause.'[38] The body had been laid unsalted in an upper room of a pub, and the fat around the omentum flowed through Wharton's fingers during the first incision. However Wharton's curiousity had overcome his nausea at the body and allowed him to act with dispassion when trying to ascertain the cause of plague. He was part of the emotional community of medical men who had been trained to act in situations that normally would provoke disgust and even fear. They emulated their teachers in anatomy who instilled fascination, awe and a strong desire to learn from the body. This helped them to overcome the sight and smell of a cadaver. Harvey's remark, 'I have forgotten many things' refers to this training. The desire for knowledge could temporarily suspend disgust but not permanently wipe out the memory of the smell, touch and sight of a decaying or diseased body. With this in mind let us consider Harvey's career as an anatomist.

The making of an anatomist

On his return to England from Padua, Harvey first obtained membership in 1603 of the College of Physicians and the following year he married Elizabeth, the daughter of Dr Lancelot Browne. In marrying Elizabeth Browne, Harvey displayed his social ambition to rise above the level of a merchant's son from Folkestone, Kent.[39] Lancelot Browne was one of the court physicians to James I and appeared to have tried unsuccessfully, in 1604, to obtain for his son-in-law a position at court and an appointment as physician to the Tower of London. In 1609 as a Fellow of the College, however, Harvey was successful in gaining a position as a physician to St Bartholomew's Hospital.[40] By 1614 he was one of the Censors of the College and in 1615 accepted the post of Lumleian lecturer. This was a stipendiary position and Harvey, with some significant gaps due to the Civil War, was to hold it for 41 years. He lectured on anatomy to physicians and surgeons at the College every two years from 1616 and held a five-day dissection each winter.

Harvey followed the approach he had been taught at Padua. He focused on the function and purpose of each anatomical structure, ultimately relating it to the cause

38 From the letterbook of Thomas Wharton, quoted in Harley, David (July 1994) 'Political Post-mortems and Morbid Anatomy in Seventeenth-Century England', *Social History of Medicine*, 7 (1), pp. 1–28.

39 See Aubrey, pp. 129–32.

40 He received an annual stipend of £25 and 'was required to attend on at least one day a week in the Great Hall of the Hospital to see his patients and prescribe for them, and to come at any other time at the request of the Matron. He was to write his prescriptions in a book without favour or gain to himself. He was expected to go to the wards only if the patient was too ill to come to him.' He also supervised the surgeons. See Medvei, Victor Cornelius and Thornton, John L. (1974), *The Royal Hospital of Saint Bartholomew 1123–1973*, London: The Royal Hospital of Saint Bartholomew, p. 105.

of disease rather than describing and enumerating the parts.[41] Under the heading *Canons of General Anatomy* Harvey detailed the first four principles according to which the anatomy and surgery lessons were to be conducted:

> 1. Shew as much in one viewing as can be, from the whole belly or from the whole of some other part ... .
> 2. Point out the peculiarities of the particular body ... and the things that are new or but newly discovered.
> 3. To supplye only by speech what cannot be shewn, on your own credit or by authority.
> 4. Cutt up as much as may be in the view of all, that practical skill may be learned together with theoretical knowledge.[42]

Like all novice medical men Harvey learned that it was the quickly decaying cadaver that dictated the timing and contents of the dissection. But given these restrictions Harvey was obviously determined to individualise each lesson, allowing the 'peculiarities' of the body to guide his presentation and yet still retain control of the dissecting process. For him the body was not a stable object but one that was constantly changing in terms of decaying tissues, diseases it might reveal and smells it emanated.

Harvey's *Canons* reflected the qualities necessary in a skilled anatomist: faithful eyes to see and show the body, an eloquent tongue to speak of the strangeness of this body and relate it to new knowledge, a keen mind able to explain what cannot be seen, and a sharp knife to cut up the body for the best viewing by the audience. This is the low style anatomy if we use Klestinec's definition, oriented around dissection, structural anatomy and the students, but it also contains elements of the high style in Harvey's desire to promote the symbolic significance of anatomy and the anatomist.

No first-hand accounts or illustrations of Harvey conducting his anatomies at the Royal College of Physicians in London are known to exist. Luke Wilson has attempted to reconstruct Harvey's personal lecture notes from the second decade of the seventeenth century, 'as a text that was written obviously but more subtly too, in his response to the claims the body lays to the attentions of the mind.'[43] The *Prelectiones anatomiae universalis* date from about 1616 to 1626, and Wilson argues that in them Harvey can be viewed as reconstituting the body 'analogically, in the tension between the absolute difference between anatomist and cadaver.'[44] By this Wilson means that over time the corpse is first ritually dismantled through the dissection and then reconstituted through the anatomy. In dissecting, the anatomist demonstrates that the body is dead and, by contrast, highlights the animation of

41 See Cunningham, Andrew (1997), *The Anatomical Renaissance: The Resurrection of the Anatomical Projects of the Ancients*, Aldershot: Scolar Press.

42 Whitteridge, p. 16.

43 Wilson, Luke (Winter, 1987) 'William Harvey's *Prelectiones*: The Performance of the Body in the Renaissance Theater of Anatomy, *Representations*, 17, pp. 62–95, quotation from p. 62. From the dating Harvey obviously emended his lectures with successive anatomies and included notes to remind himself to change the format of particular passages in the future. Also see Whitteridge, pp. 88–104.

44 Ibid., p. 89.

the spectators and the anatomist. Wilson concludes that showing the morbidity of the cadaver made conscious to the spectators that their bodies were healthy.[45] Through anatomy Harvey managed his own anxiety and that of the audience. As Jonathon Sawday also concludes, Wilson argues that dissection was a ritual act of public revilement and identification-in-difference, a repetition of the execution that preceded it and provided the body that was to be its subject.[46]

Wilson is less convincing when he describes the anatomy (as opposed to the preliminary dissection) as:

> ... the reversal in fantasy both of the dissection and of the execution that preceded it, a retroactive pardoning of the guilty that repairs the damage that the punisher in his punishment, and the anatomist in his dissection; have inadvertently worked against themselves. Here, therefore, is the romance of reanimation to balance against the tragedy of dismemberment.[47]

This interpretation ignores the fact that many of Harvey's anatomical experiences did not come from dissecting unknown criminals but from performing post-mortems on patients, often intimately known and even related to him.[48]

A different portrayal of Harvey as lecturer is presented by Robert Erickson. He sees Harvey as possessing a vivid sense of theatre, both of himself as a public performer and of the theatre of the body which he opened to perform upon:

> Harvey seems not unlike an Old Testament priest reincarnated, cutting up sheep, goats, female deer, and a variety of other animals (occasionally practising vivisection) as sacrifices to a new goddess, Truth. As an anatomist-author, Harvey was recreating in his finite capacity the divine role of the original anatomist-Author of humankind in Genesis 2 who dissected Adam in order to create a new human being, Eve.[49]

As Thomas Baines had written of Molinetti at Padua, 'thus you do not display yourself, the anatomist, but what is far greater, God.'

While Erickson focuses upon *De motu cordis* rather than the *Prelectiones*, his analysis of the former as, 'a kind of travel narrative of what happens inside the body ... an anatomical labyrinth' is relevant to the latter. Reading the *Prelectiones* is akin to traversing the map of the body. In short phrases Harvey carefully builds an oral, visual and an olfactory portrait of the body gone awry, illustrating each point of the function of the parts with some personal observation of his own. Essentially he speaks for the voiceless organs:

---

45 *Idem.*

46 *Idem.*

47 Ibid., p. 90. Also see Sawday, *The Body Emblazoned,* particularly the first chapter.

48 Keele, 'William Harvey as Morbid Anatomist', p. 678.

49 Erickson, Robert A. (1993), 'William Harvey's *De motu cordis* and "The Republick of Literature,"' in Roberts, Marie Mulvey, and Porter, Roy (eds), *Literature and Medicine During the Eighteenth Century*, London and New York: Routledge, pp. 58–83, quotation from p. 61.

> Size of the stomach. Stomachs of certain gluttons. Gourmandisers, drinkers, have been of huge capacity; many ancient and recent accounts [of these] ... WH Wilkinson of Cambridg. Pigg of ye spitt ... . Sometimes they [testicles] are swollen with a very great quantity of water and flatus; the man behind covent garden bigger than his belly; forme, penis as if of a buffalo ... . I know a Paduan capable of coitus with the glans removed ... . Substance [of the bladder is] membranous, white, and sinewy for strength and retention. Wherefore if wounded it does not consolidate except in the neck, as we have seen daily in dissection; especially in children, torn not cutt. [50]

By interweaving anatomical and salacious knowledge, Harvey was keeping his audience's attention and giving them a vivid moving picture of the interior of the body. As they travelled from stomach to penis to bladder, the *Prelectiones* acted as a tour guide of the major sights along the way.

Unfortunately little evidence has been found of the reception of Harvey's lectures in anatomy and surgery. A rare exception is a Dr Peter Browne (1575–1624) who published a pamphlet *Pseudo-medicorum anatomia* in 1624 with Latin verses praising some of the Fellows of the College. The verses are addressed to the President and Fellows of the College and include one on Harvey. As Geoffrey Keynes notes, Browne 'could have heard Harvey lecture on many occasions over a period of seven years and the date of his book (1624) ensures that his opinion was not influenced by Harvey's later fame after the publication of *De motu cordis* in 1628'[51]:

> They talk of your learnedly and skilfully treating of anatomy. I have seen it, and your dexterity is hardly to be matched. Your reading is most learned, your dissecting marvellous.

50 *The Anatomical Lectures*, pp. 85, 140 and 149. Ralph Wilkinson (*c.*1544–1609) was a fellow of the College of Physicians and preceded Harvey as Physician to St Bartholomew's Hospital. His 'prowess at the table' would therefore be well known to Harvey and his students. Many of Harvey's writings were destroyed by Parliamentary troops in 1642 when his apartments in the Palace of Whitehall were raided 'lost ... to the prejudice (I may boldly say it) of the Commonwealth of Learning', as Harvey phrased it in *De generatione* in 1653, Keynes, *Life*, p.162. However remaining notes for *De motu locali animalium*, 1627, echo the language of his lecture notes and mention family members, 'risus sardonicus, uncle William Halke dying.' Keynes, *Life*, p. 165.

51 Keynes, *Life*, p. 110.

> What then? Does your skilled hand make me bold? It has! and I should wish (for this your deeds deserve)That what my Muse does first, your clever hand should then cut up.[52]

The references to Harvey's dexterity, reading, dissecting and skilled hand echoes the *Canons* of his lectures. The effect on Peter Browne was to fill him with courage when it came to dissecting and perhaps cutting on patients.

Harvey's fascination with the monstrous and salacious body extended to the patients he chose, or in some cases, was ordered to see. As a Royal Physician he oversaw the interrogation of witches, examined a nobleman with a hole in his chest through which the beating heart could be touched and performed an autopsy on 'Old Parr', reputed to be 152 years old at the time of his death. As a London physician Harvey appears to have specialized to some extent in obstetric and gynaecologic cases. Some of these have been preserved in *De generatione animalium*, a book published in 1651 to showcase Harvey's work on animal reproduction.

Harvey was named by Charles I to direct an examination by surgeons and midwives of four alleged witches from Lancashire in 1634. No incriminating marks of the devil were found, such as extra nipples to succour familiars or marks of the devil, and the women were released. Perhaps Harvey was chosen by the king to manage the search of the women's bodies because of his interest in obstetric and gynaecological cases and the common belief that marks of witchcraft were typically hidden in women's *secret parts*. Another mark of witchcraft was insensitivity to pain. Robert Boyle recalled Mr Hollyer, a lithotomist at St Thomas' Hospital, describing Harvey's interest in Mary, 'a Maid of about eighteen Years of age, who ... had so lost the sense of feeling in the external parts of her Body' that Hollyer could pin a handkerchief to her neck and cause no pain. 'Dr. Harvey, out of Curiosity, visited her sometimes; and suspecting her strange Distemper to be chiefly Uterine and curable onely by *Hymeneal* Exercises, he advised her Parents ... to take her home, and provide her a Husband ... to many Mens wonder.'[53] Mary was not magical, just hysterical.

Harvey was also the arbiter of truth in two other famous cases. Thomas Howard, the Earl of Arundel brought Thomas Parr to London from one of his Shropshire estates to meet the king on account of Parr having reportedly reached the age of 152. Parr soon died, and Harvey was ordered to perform an autopsy on behalf of

---

52 Ibid., pp.110–111. Keynes gives the Latin and the translation.

> *Doctori* Harvey
> TE dextrè & doctè Anatomen tractare loquuntur:
> Vidi, & dexteritas vix imitanda tua est.
> Lectio perdocta est, dissectio mira: quid ergò?
> nùm tua me audacem dextera docta facit?
> Fecit, & optarem, nam sic tua facta merentur,
> ut quae *Musa priùs*, post tua dextra secet.

Also see, Rowe, Katherine, '"God's handy worke": Divine Complicity and the Anatomist's Touch', in Hillman, David and Mazzio, Carlo (eds) (1997), *The Body In Parts: Fantasies of Corporeality in Early Modern*, London and New York: Routledge, pp. 284–309.

53 Keynes, *Life*, p. 212.

Charles I. The report of the autopsy of 'Old Parr' at the age of 152 begins with Harvey noting that 'the dissection of his dead body' took place on Queen Henrietta Maria's birthday, 16 November 1635. This gift was perhaps the most unusual one the queen received that year. Harvey diagnosed the cause of death as suffocation due to the filthy air of London. In Shropshire's 'clean, rarefied, coolish and circulating air' Parr's diaphragm and lungs had been freely inflated and deflated. His rich diet in London also led to a 'less vigorous circulation of the blood'.[54] Harvey was the expert on this topic after all and the report is notable for its focus on the blood, the heart and the genitalia. The latter interest was due to reports that Old Parr had intercourse with his wife up to the age of 140. Harvey was able to confirm that the fine condition of the genital organs suggested that this was in fact true.

Around 1640 King Charles I heard of the case of Viscount Hugh Montgomery, who had a plate covering a large opening in his thorax as a result of a fall when a child. Harvey visited him to ascertain the truth of the matter. His excitement was evident on discovering that he could feel the beating heart through the opening:

> Where I presently beheld a vast hole in his breast, into which I could easily put my three Fore-fingers and my Thumb: and at the first entrance I perceived a certain fleshy part sticking out, which was driven in and out by reciprocal motion ... . Being now amazed at the novelty of the thing, I search it again and again ... (and laying one hand upon his wrest, and the other upon his heart) ... . I concluded it to be no part of the Lungs, but the Cone or Substance of the heart.[55]

Harvey brought Montgomery to the king so he could 'see, and handle this strange and singular Accident with his own Senses; namely, the Heart and its Ventricles in their pulsation, in a young and sprightly Gentleman, without offense to him. Whereupon the King himself consented with me, That the Heart is deprived of the Sense of Feeling.'[56] Charles I became Harvey's student, his eyes were directed, his hands were guided and the examination of Montgomery resulted in an anatomical truth – the heart is insensible. The case was included in Harvey's *De generatione animalium*.

The three Lancashire witches, along with Mary the Maid, Old Parr and Montgomery, show Harvey's diligence as an anatomist and his belief that examining bodies allowed one to establish the truth. The witches were found to be falsely accused, Mary had a uterine disorder, Old Parr died of suffocation and bad circulation, Montgomery was not a fraud but a wonder. The cases also reveal Harvey's sceptical attitude towards written or verbal accounts of the unusual or the inexplicable and his need to put such accounts to test through cutting, seeing and training others to see the truth in the body. Did such skill in anatomy actually make one a better doctor? Many were doubtful. Even John Aubrey, the Wiltshire natural philosopher who knew Harvey first hand and thought of himself as one of his friends stated:

---

54 Ibid., p. 224. The report was written in Latin and given to Dr John Betts by Michael Harvey, William Harvey's nephew. Betts published it as a postscript to *De ortu et natura sanguinis*, (1669), London.

55 Keynes, *Life*, p.156.

56 *Idem*.

> All his Profession would allow him to be an excellent Anatomist, but I never heard of any that admired his Therapeutique way. I knew severall practisers in London that would not have given 3d. for one of his Bills; and that a man could hardly tell by one of his Bills what he did aime at.[57]

The value of anatomy in the practice of medicine

On 1 July 1651 Viscount Conway wrote a letter to his daughter-in-law Anne Conway. Anne suffered from violent and painful headaches:

> I heare that you have a great opinion of Doctor Harvey. I thinke you doe well to love and respect a person of his merite for I thinke he hath deserved extreamely well of all learned men, for what he hath found out, or offered to the world to enquire farther into: he is a most excelent Anatomist, and I conceive that to be his Masterpiece, which knowledge is many times of very great use in consultations, but in the practicke of Physicke I conceive him to be mutch, many times, governed by his Phantasy ... to have a Physitian abound in phantasie is a very perilous thing, occations in diseases are very often suddaine, therefore one ought to have a Physitian that should be governed only by his judgment ... [58]

What did the Viscount mean by 'Phantasy'? Perhaps a further letter to Anne Conway just a few months later in December 1651 may help answer this. This time it was from John Finch, the aforementioned medical student at Padua, who was also Anne's brother:

> I was on Saturday with Sir Kenelm Digby [in Paris] where I had some philosophicall discourse: and he heard of your marriage, but wondered with me at your story of Dr Harvey. I must confesse I have scarce faith enough to believe he would cutt himself but rather believe he voyded that stone you speake of then cutt it out; for I doe not see it was possible for him in two days to be able to goe abroad otherwise.[59]

What does this tell us of the reputation of William Harvey?[60] Finch's disbelief in the story of Harvey operating on himself for a bladder stone seems predicated on the notion that Harvey would not have been walking around a mere two days after

57 Aubrey, p. 132. A Bill was a prescription.

58 Keynes, *Life*, p. 393. Anne Conway was Heneage Finch's step-sister. John Finch also wrote to his sister in August 1652 wondering at Harvey's 'little successe' in her case. p. 394.

59 Nicolson, Marjorie Hope, (ed.) (1930), *Conway Letters: The Correspondence of Anne, Viscountess Conway, Henry More, and their Friends,1642–1684*, New Haven: Yale University Press, p. 60. Nicolson noted that this story appeared nowhere else.

60 Some stories linger on into contemporary times. Antonia Fraser (1973) states that at the battle of Edgehill on 23 October 1642, 'William Harvey, the scientist, who read a book under a hedge until a bullet grazed the ground, literally showed *sangfroid* by pulling a dead body over him for warmth against the cold clear weather of that freezing night.' *Cromwell, Our Chief of Men*, London: Weidenfeld and Nicolson, p. 96. However she provides no citation for this story and I have not been able to find it elsewhere. It probably is a confusion with the story of Sir Gervase Scrope. Harvey told John Aubrey that Scrope had been left for dead on the field, stripped of his belongings, and woke to find his bleeding stopped by the cold in the

the operation, rather than on the fact that he would not have 'cutt himself' to begin with.

Such stories regarding the bizarre and 'phantastical' nature of those who dissected for a living were beginning to circulate in early modern Europe. Beginning in the 1530s a haze of unsavoury stories on the topic of vivisection gradually collected around the names of famous anatomists.[61] Anatomical authors were willing to boast of their illicit behaviours in procuring cadavers and so fan the rumours of vivisection. It was Vesalius who marks the real turning point:

> One of the most surprising aspects of his great treatise *On the Fabric of the Human Body* (1543) compared to the works of his predecessors, is his lack of respect for persons and his candid pride in the acts of daring and deception required to obtain what he considered an adequate supply of cadavers. He and his students forged keys, rifled tombs and gibbets, and stole in and out of ossuaries in a series of nighttime escapades that he recounts with evident relish and amusement ...[62]

Similarly the young Felix Platter gleefully recounted his role in 'every secret autopsy of corpses' while a medical student at Montpellier in 1554. He referred to the repulsion 'I had felt at first' when I came 'to put my own hand to the scalpel' but admitted this quickly passed.[63] Soon Platter could aid in the grave robbing and dissection of a 'student we had known'. Yet as with Harvey the smell of rotting organs lingered long in Platter's memory, 'the lungs were decomposed and stank horribly, despite the vinegar that we sprinkled on them ...'[64]

A hundred years after Vesalius the Danish Royal anatomist Thomas Bartholin still found the career of a dissector filled with trials and tribulations:

> Neither in our age nor any former one will you readily find an eminent anatomist who has placed domestic ease before the rigors of travel, although it must be warned that the goal sought will not always be a happy one .... Hence almost everywhere anatomists have been victims of misfortune, and if some have been able to avoid these snares that have been debilitated by the stench of the cadavers so that few can hope to reach a venerable age .... Finally, if spared, they complete the journey and grow old at home with Galen, with no reward except wearied and bloody hands, and those empty.[65]

Here was the anatomist as hero and martyr with his 'wearied and bloody hands', scorned by his fellow countrymen and destined to live out his life in poverty. The

---

middle of the night and 'was faine to drawe a dead body upon him for warmeth-sake.' Harvey treated him after Scrope's son recovered him from the battlefield. Keynes, *Life*, p. 290.

61 Park, Katherine (1994), 'The Criminal and Saintly Body: Autopsy and Dissection in Renaissance Italy', *Renaissance Quarterly*. 47, pp. 1–33.

62 Ibid., p. 17.

63 *Beloved Son Felix: The Journal of Felix Platter a medical student at Montpellier in the Sixteenth Century* (1961), trans. and introduced by Jennett, Sean, London: Frederick Muller Limited, p. 89.

64 Ibid., p. 90.

65 Bartholin, Thomas (1961), *On the Burning of His Library and On Medical Travel*, trans. O'Malley, C.D., Lawrence: The University of Kansas Libraries, p. 52.

elderly Bartholin had forgotten or perhaps never experienced the excitement of a night-time hunt for cadavers. However he recalled the stench of the cadavers and related this to the premature deaths of some anatomists. This was an argument that grew in strength throughout the next two centuries. Bartholin also drew attention to the misunderstanding that those who dissected were subject to, and echoed Harvey's words that many perceived him to be 'crack-brain'd' due to his reliance on anatomy as truth.

Certainly the gruesome yet fascinating art of anatomy had an effect upon the emotions of others. In 1627 or 1628 Joseph Mede, a divinity student at Christ's College Cambridge, described a dissection in a letter to his father:

> We had an anatomy lecture upon a boy of some 18 years old, Monday, Tuesday, Wednesday, twise a day the last two dayes. I was once there, but saw it so ill accommodated that I came no more; for it was in the regent house upon a table, when onlye halfe a skore doctors could come to see anything, standing close by the table, and so hindering others seeing, which was the chiefe; for I can read as good as they could heare, and with more ease. It will be next time I hope better, for our new doctor will have one every yeare. We heare talke that the body was begged before any was condemned, which if true was very absurd.[66]

Mede was about the age of the boy who had been hanged but here he expresses no emotion except for frustration. He hopes that there will be another opportunity where he can see the body rather than just hear the lecture. He finds it ludicrous that this body may have been preordered by the anatomist, and the whole event strikes Mede as somewhat farcical with the crowd of doctors around the table shoving and pushing one another in an attempt to see the dissection.

On 16 April 1631 Mede stumbled across the remains of a dissected cadaver and this time he had a different reaction. He wrote home to his father about the shock it gave him:

> Going on Wednesday from Jesus Colledge pensionary with Dr Ward to his Colledge through the closes and gardens and espying a garden dore open I entred and saw there a hideous sight of the skull and all the other bones of a man with ligaments and tendons hanging and drying in the sun by strings upon trees, etc., I asked what it meant. They told me it was the pedler they anatomised this Lent and that when his bones were dry they were to sett together again as they did naturally and so reserved in a chest or coffin for their use who desired such an inspection. It was the garden of one Seale a surgeon and a chief in dissection.[67]

Unlike the anatomy lecture, this event was unexpected and Mede was initially bewildered by it, 'I asked what it meant.'

---

66 Keynes, *Life*, p. 16.

67 Costello, William T. (1958), *The Scholastic Curriculum at Early Seventeenth-Century Cambridge*, Cambridge, MA: Harvard University Press, p. 130. Costello speculates that the dissector was perhaps the Regius Professor of Physic, John Collins (1572–1634) who was also lecturer in anatomy to the College of Physicians.

From Conway's story of Harvey cutting on himself for the stone, to Platter stealing corpses and retching at the smell of decay, to Bartholin's plaintive lament that anatomists get no respect, to Mede's shock at seeing an eviscerated carcass hanging from the trees in a university garden, the evidence of the development of an unsavoury reputation for those who dissected mounted. At the same time the qualities desired in an anatomist were being defined and satirized.

The focus of much of the doggerel was the masculine bravery – or lack thereof – of certain dissectors. In Oxford Dr Thomas Clayton (1575–1647) arranged for his eldest son, Thomas (1612–93), to succeed him as the Tomlins reader in anatomy. He was clearly unsuited for these posts, 'being posses'd with a timorous and effeminate Humour, [he] could never endure the sight of a mangled or bloody Body.'[68] Clayton lacked all the qualities necessary to be a good anatomist as outlined by Harvey. He could not 'shew, cutt or point out' any of the marvels or monstrosities of nature. In turn his own body was declared to be monstrous because he had the humoral makeup of a woman. Poor Thomas Clayton was naturally subjected to scurrilous student songs:

Well noble Knight our Anatomiste
Take my advice.
Bee pleas'd to desist from reading.
And mistake no parte
No not a liver for the hart
As last you did.
Trade not in blood
Be advised by your friends,
o good Sr Thomas.[69]

William Petty (1623–87), the son of a Romsey, Kent clothier and graduate in medicine of Leiden University deputized for the squeamish Thomas Clayton. As one of the early admirers of Harvey's accomplishments, Petty had already undertaken anatomical research in Paris and London during the late 1640s. As with Harvey, there soon arose a mythology surrounding Petty as an anatomist of some bravado, skill and imagination. According to John Aubrey, 'Anatomy was then but little understood by the university, and I remember he [Petty] kept a body that he brought by water from Reding a good while to read upon some way soused or pickled.'[70] In contrast to Thomas Clayton's lack of courage when faced with a corpse, the story of William Petty's role in the resuscitation of Anne Greene in 1650 was one of drama and heroics.[71]

---

68 Dewhurst, Kenneth (1980), *Willis' Oxford Lectures*, Oxford: Sandford Publications, p. 402. Clayton was a devout Royalist, the Master of Pembroke College and had succeeded his father-in-law to the post of Regius Professor. The quotation regarding Clayton's son comes from Anthony á Wood (1721), *Athenae Oxonienses*, 2nd ed., 2, p. 807.

69 Dewhurst, p. 403.

70 Ibid., p. 404. In 1651 Petty left Oxford to serve as Physician-in-Chief to Cromwell's army in Ireland.

71 Scott Mandelbrote gives a complete and intriguing account of this incident in (2005), 'William Petty and Anne Greene: Medical and Political Reform in Commonwealth Oxford' in

Her tale was published as a broadsheet by a Richard Watkins in Oxford with the catchy title of *Newes from the Dead. Or a true and Exact Narration of the Miraculous deliverance of Anne Greene* (1651). A servant girl, Greene was found guilty of murdering her illegitimate child, and on the 14 December 1650 she was publicly hanged in the centre of Oxford. Petty had made arrangements with the authorities to take her body to his High Street lodgings. It was also the home of John Clarke who had been Harvey's apothecary. There he was to dissect her with the aid of Thomas Willis (1621–75) in front of members of an experimental club that met weekly in his rooms.[72]

Anne Greene hung for nearly half an hour and, as was customary, her friends swung on her legs to speed her death. The undersheriff began to fear that they would pull the rope and her body down and quickly ordered the rope to be cut and her body placed in a coffin, provided by Petty. This was part of the fee he had paid for the opportunity to dissect her. When the coffin was opened at Petty's lodgings, however, Anne Greene was heard to breathe with a rattling noise, and no doubt in terror at her suffering more, an onlooker stamped several times on her chest and stomach to try to kill her.

When Petty and Willis entered the room they were told she appeared to have recently taken a breath and noticed that she 'rattle againe where-upon wee fell to worke'.[73] Greene was placed in Petty's bed, hot cordials were poured down her throat, she was bled, given a clyster, her feet and hands were vigorously rubbed, a feather was put down her throat and a woman obligingly rolled into bed to help warm her. The following morning she was talking rationally, and a delighted Petty and Willis sat down to write and submit a petition for mercy. There was no law that said she could not be hanged again, and the ground of their appeal was that her abortive or stillborn foetus had been imperfect and therefore not viable. After obtaining a pardon, Petty and Willis exhibited Greene as a medical curiosity in her coffin in the very room where they would have dissected her. Greene's father was brought in to collect the entrance fees and they had to arrange for guards to control the multitudes that flocked to see her. Petty and Willis were celebrated in verse and prose, including these lines from an undergraduate of Christ Church:

> Thus 'tis more easy to recall the Dead
> Than to restore a once-lost Maidenhead.[74]

Anne Green lived another nine years, married and had three children. As Mandelbrote demonstrates, Petty was careful to construct the revival of Anne Greene as a consequence of his understanding of blood circulation and willingness to experiment,

---

The Practice of Reform in Health, Medicine, and Science, 1500–2000, pp. 125–49.

72 Ibid., p. 125.

73 Ibid., p. 126 quoting from a letter to Samuel Hartlib written by Petty on 16 December 1650.

74 Watkins includes the verse in 1651, *Newes from the Dead. Or a true and Exact Narration of the Miraculous deliverance of Anne Greene*, Oxford, and states the author was Kingsmill Lucy, p. 9. Petty gave his version of Anne Greene's recovery. See (1927), *The Petty Papers*, Marquis of Lansdowne (ed.), London, 2, pp. 157–67. Robert Plot in (1677), *The*

rather than providence. It made Petty's reputation and fortune as a cool-headed and skilled anatomist.[75]

On a more serious note, elegies were composed reflecting the character of those who anatomized. In 1677 Nathaniel Williams published an elegy for Thomas Willis, one of Anne Greene's revivers. Its portrayal of the wonders anatomists reveal, and the final anatomy their own bodies make, echo the mixture of unease and fascination for dissection seen by the public of the period:

> Thou knew the wonderous art,
> And order of each part ...
> In the whole lump, how every sense,
> Contributes to the health's defense.
> The severall, Channels which convey,
> The vitall current every way,
> Trackst wise Nature every where,
> In every region, every sphere,
> Fathomest the mistery
> Of deepe Anathomy.
> The unactive carcasse thou hadst preyed upon,
> And stript it to a sceleton,
> But now alas! the art is gone,
> And now on thee,
> The crawling Worms experience their Anatomy.[76]

The references in Willis's elegy to the relentless and predatory nature of anatomists – and the ultimate futility of such detailed knowledge of the corruptible body – were not lost on the critics of dissection-crazed physicians. Perhaps reflective of the fact that the Royalist Harvey's programme of sustained anatomizing was taking hold, wholesale attacks on the art of anatomy were launched during the Interregnum as part of the campaigns to reform medicine.

In *Matacotechnia medicinae praxeos:the Vanity of the Craft of Physick* (1651) the self-avowed 'Chymiatrophilos' Noah Biggs attacked the cruelty and uselessness of anatomy. He made particular reference to William Harvey and his followers 'who inquire unto capillary veins':

> To what ends tends the Anatomy of these two thousand years, with those tedious lectures, if the sanation of diseases, be not more happier at this day, then of old? What meanes that tearing and Cadaverous dissection of bodies, with that curious inspection and inquisition into the capillary veines, if we may not learn by the Errors of the Ancients, and if we may not make an emendation of those things that are past.[77]

Natural History of Oxfordshire, Oxford, p. 47, mentions Greene's supposedly spotless later years.

75 Mandelbrote, 'William Petty and Anne Greene: Medical and Political Reform in Commonwealth Oxford', p. 147

76 Aubrey, p. 176.

77 Noah Biggs, *Mataeotechnia medicinae*: *The vanity of the craft of physick; or, A new dispensatory* ... London, 1651, p. 9. Biggs's true identity has never been established; however, see Cook, Harold J. (1986), *The Decline of the Old Medical Regime in Stuart London*, Ithaca

For Biggs dissecting led not to new medical knowledge but to new deaths:

> For there is nothing more hard, more inhumane and full of Cruelty, among all *humane Arts*, through so many ages undertaken and usurp'd then that art, which by a concentrick subscription doth make new experiments by the deaths of men where the Earth covers the vices, the errors & frauds of its professors ...[78]

The London physician Gideon Harvey (no relation to William) wrote a savage satire of the monopoly of the College of Physicians in 1683 entitled *The Conclave of Physicians, Detecting their Intrigues, Frauds, and Plots, Against their Patients.* In it he compared anatomy to the practice of cannibalism.[79] Gideon Harvey referred to the College as the 'Conclave of Physicians to the Venetians', thus managing in one fell swoop to attack English physicians in particular and Roman Catholicism in general:

> Their immolations are celebrated chiefly in the *Winter* upon Dogs and Cats by the younger fry, and sometimes upon humane bodies performed by the Hangman, their subservient Officer, which being conveyed to their *Chauncel*, the *Cardinals* in their turn fall hewing and slaying these Carcases like *Cannibals*, to the intent all Spectators (to whom at such *Festivals* free egress and regress is granted) may behold them sitting in their *Pontisicalibus*, and making a pretended narrower search into the parts of mans body, insinuating thereby to these gazers their incomparable Skill and Learning, not without a plain *Innuendo*, that they should send for them in time of Sickness ... .[80]

Gideon Harvey bitterly concluded that the illusion of anatomy being the road to medical progress was created to attract customers. Anatomists created public displays

---

and London: Cornell University Press. Cook explains that Biggs's work 'was addressed to the Parliament, which, Biggs said, had been directed by Cromwell to undertake the reform of all the professions', p. 122. Debus, Allen G. 'Paracelsian Medicine: Noah Biggs and the Problem of Medical Reform', in Debus, Allen G. (ed.) (1974), *Medicine in Seventeenth Century England*, Berkeley: University of California Press, pp. 33–48, describes Biggs as a devout Iatrochemist who believed that God creates and chooses true physicians not men, or universities.

78 Biggs, p. 14.

79 Gideon Harvey (1640?–1700?) was born in Holland, son of John and Elizabeth Harvey. He studied medicine, botany and anatomy at Leiden and Paris and probably obtained his MD and MB at a minor French university. He settled in London after the Restoration and in 1675 he became physician-in-ordinary to Charles II. In 1683 he published *The Conclave of Physicians*, supposedly set in Paris, attacking the College of Physicians. The same year Harvey was satirised in a thirty-page work, *Gideon's Fleece, or The Sieur de Frisk, an heroick Poem. Written on the cursory perusal of a late Book call'd The Conclave of Physicians by a Friend to the Muses*. Harvey was made physician of the Tower by William and Mary. Opinions of Gideon Harvey's works have been poor. Gideon Harvey rather than Christopher Merrett most likely wrote *The Accomplisht Physician, the Honest apothecary, and the skilful Chyrurgeon*, 1670.

80 Harvey, Gideon (1683), *The Conclave of Physicians,* London, 'The Introduction', p. 8.

only on safe bodies, those dead and therefore incurable, rather than the living and in pain. No wonder they were so successful at marketing themselves.[81]

In *The Art of Curing Diseases by Expectation* (1669) he ultimately attacked the father of anatomy himself. Gideon Harvey claimed that William Harvey's anatomical proficiency did not guarantee his therapeutic skills; in fact, they guaranteed his lack of them. As evidence he gave details of a number of cases where William Harvey had wrongly diagnosed or wrongly prescribed:

> ... one Mr. Farwell, Barrister of the Temple, was Patient and Complainent of a painful disease in his belly ... Dr. Harvey ingrossed to himself the speaking part (a noisy 'Consult' of doctors were present) by reason of his extraordinary claim to Anatomy ... after a long contrectation of all the abdomen, did very magisterially and positively assert all his symptoms to arise from an Aneurism of an artery, and therefore incurable, as being too remote to come at, wherein all, except Dr. Bates, very readily concur'd, though it was a most absurd offer in opinion, as I ever yet heard.[82]

Gideon Harvey concluded that Harvey's practical mismanagement of cases stemmed from hubris based upon his knowledge of vivisecting animals:[83]

> No doubt but Dr. Harvey in Anatomy, and happiness of theoretic discoveries might justly pretend the precedency of all his contemporaries; and others before and since have also arrived to a great proficiency in cat and dog-cutting, also calf-head and sheeps-pluck dissecting; yet few of 'em when concerne in practice, were gifted with sagacity to know diseases when offered to their view, much less capable of curing them; in which curative particular the thinking Physician has the advantage, though the prating Physician by his pretended Anatomy ingrosses the opinion of mankind.[84]

For Noah Biggs and Gideon Harvey, anatomy was a 'prating art' much like quackery where practitioners dazzled the public with sleight of hand and empty rhetoric. Yet there was also a more serious accusation concerning the fundamental inhumanity of any physician who has learned to 'do no harm' to his patients through long training in dissection and vivisection.

Everyone agreed that William Harvey was an excellent anatomist but that is as far as the agreement appears to have gone. He never lost an opportunity to dissect and bemoaned when none presented itself:

81 For more on Gideon Harvey and other critics of William Harvey's discovery of the circulation of the blood, see Frank, 'The Image of Harvey in Commonwealth and Restoration England', in *William Harvey and His Age,* pp. 103–43, especially pp.132–3.

82 Harvey, *The Conclave*, p. 17.

83 Ibid., p. 180.

84 *Memorials of Harvey*, Aveling, J.H.(ed.) (1875), London: J. & A. Churchill, p. 17. The quotation is taken from Gideon Harvey (1689), *The Art of Curing Diseases by Expectation,* London, Chapter XXII.

> ... I can only complayne, that by the waye we could scarce see a dogg crow kite Raven or any bird, or any thinge to anatomise only sum few miserable people the reliques of the war & the plague where famine had made anatomies before I came.[85]

Harvey expressed himself as a medical man by using the language of a dissector and vivisector. A poor laundress came to see him with a prolapsed uterus:[86]

> ... as large as a Bulls Cod, dangling between her leggs: so that I suspected that, not onely the sheath, but that the womb it selfe was now inverted, or else that she was diseased with a Uterine hernia, or Rupture. It grew at last bigger than a mans head, being then a hard tumour, and hanging downe to her knees did much pain her, so that she could not goe (but upon all foure) and breaking just in the bottom of it, it did effund a moisture (as if it had been an Ulcer) and blood with it. [87]

He collected specimens from the living and the dead, be they family members or patients, and exhibited them to his friends:

> But the following night, an Infant perfectly shaped, of a span long, was cast out of that Tumour, but it was dead; and the next morning thay brought it to me; which having embowelled, I kept swimming in cold water without corruption for some moneths time, shewing it to many of my friends (as a miraculous spectacle.)[88]

Harvey remembered what he saw and tried to forget what he smelt:

> **WH** I saw it [the bladder] ulcerated in lues venerea through the whole internal region for years, the kidney intact; the thick, fleshy bladder, as a matrix for it, internally *like vnshorne velvet livid* gangrenous with fetid, disturbed and purulent urines.[89]

He reminded his students and colleagues that not only was anatomy fascinating, it also led to medical progress. What was seen could be cured:

---

85 Harvey was so moved by the sight of such misery and desolation that he ended his letter with ‘It is time to leave fighting when there is nothing to eat ... .’ Letter, of probably 1631, from Harvey to Viscount Dorchester, Principal Secretary to Charles I. Harvey probably travelled to France, Italy and Spain with the Duke of Lenox from 1631–32. Aveling, p. 8. Keynes, *Life,* speculates that the undated letter was written in 1630 to Dorchester, p. 193.

86 ‘One cannot overestimate the degree to which the uterus is not only called the "Sink or Common-Shoar, whereunto the rest of the parts of the Body disburden themselves" but is likewise the repository for most explanations of pathology advanced by medicine about women.’ Quoting Lazare Rivière or Riverius, (1672), *The Practice of Physick*, comp. and trans., Nicolas Culpeper, Abdiah Cole, and William Rowland, London, p. 413.

87 Harvey, William (1653), *Anatomical Exercitations Concerning the Generation of Living Creatures, to which are added particular Discourses, of Births, and of Conceptions, etc.*, London, p. 493.

88 *Idem.*

89 Harvey, *Lectures*, p. 140.

I WH saw a prolapsed uterus and cured it.[90]

He antagonized non-anatomically minded medical men by condemning their reliance on rhetoric rather than taking up the knife and performing the nasty yet necessary work of dissection:

> Frivolous and unexperienced persons do scurvily strive to overthrow by logicall and far-fetch'd arguments, or to establish such things as are meerly to be confirm'd by Anatomical dissection, and ocular testimony. It behoves him, who ever is desirous to learn, to see any thing which is in question, if it be obvious to sense or sight, whether it be so or no, or else be bound to believe those that have made tryall, for by no other clearer or more evident certainity can he learn or be taught.[91]

The emotions elicited, repressed and expressed, during his student days at the University of Padua and later in his career as a physician to kings, shaped William Harvey. In turn he modelled the ideal anatomist that his followers sought to copy and his detractors to ridicule. He gave his admirers a certain image of the anatomist to emulate: self-possessed, hard-working, voracious when it came to seeking out opportunities to open bodies and passionate about the veracity of his findings. Harvey may not have struggled much with achieving dispassion in the face of the more revolting aspects of his art, but this was not necessarily the case for those who came after him.

90 *Idem.* This may have been the poor laundress's uterus.

91 Harvey, William (1995), *The Anatomical Exercises: De Motu Cordis and De Circulatione Sanguinis in English Translation*, ed. Keynes, Geoffrey, New York: Dover Publications, p. 176. The quote is from 'Another Exercitation' in *De Circulatione Sanguinis* to Jean Riolan the Son where Harvey is refuting Riolan's objections to the circulation of the blood. Riolan was Professor of Anatomy at the University of Paris. The two essays to Riolan were published in Latin in 1649 and translated anonymously into English and published by Richard Lowndes in 1653 and 1673.

Chapter Two

Rational Minds

Our perspicacious Countryman Dr. *Harvey*, somewhere in his Book of the G*eneration of Animals*, affirms it to be no small advantage to the Brain, that Students and contemplative Men preserve their mass of Blood pure and uncorrupt.[1]

I have been driven from my Country, House, Family, Books, Friends, and Acquaintance ... My Anchors are lost, my Vessell leaks, the Winds hurry it from land, and I hourly expect to sink down-right.[2]

On 27 February 1663, 'desirous to learn',[3] Samuel Pepys made his way to the Barber-Surgeons' anatomy theatre. For a few hours he was part of the emotional community of the leading physicians and surgeons in London. After listening to the anatomy lecture by Dr Tearne on the 'kidneys, ureters, &c., which was very fine'[4] Pepys went to the Hall and enjoyed the customary banquet. Then:

After dinner, Dr. Scarborough took some of his friends and I went with them, to see the body of a lusty fellow, a seaman, that was hanged for a robbery. I did touch the body with my bare hands; it felt cold, but methought it was a very unpleasant sight ... .[5]

Having bravely touched the corpse, Pepys was far more comfortable when Scarburgh and Tearne took him to another room to see the parts that had been dissected during the lecture:

1 Charleton, Walter (1664), *A Brief Discourse Concerning the Different Wits of Men*, London, p. 51.

2 Charleton, Walter (1657), *The Immortality of the Human Soul*, London, p. 11.

3 *The Diary of Samuel Pepys*, (2001), ed. Le Gallienne, Richard, New York: The Modern Library, 2001, p. 89.

4 *Idem*. On the Hall and Anatomy theatre see, Murray, Ian and Hall, Brian, 'The Hall and the area in which we live', and Missen, John and Hill, Dennis, 'The Anatomy Theatre' in *The Company of Barbers and Surgeons* (2000), Burns, Ian (ed.), London: The Worshipful Company of Barbers, pp.45–60 and pp.111–28. The Hall burnt down in the Great Fire of 1666 but the Anatomy Theatre and Court Room were saved. In 1769 the Anatomy Theatre was demolished. Sidney Young includes a plan of the Company's Estate in Monkwell Street in *The Annals of the Barber-Surgeons of London* (1890), p. 135. He gives 1784 as the date the Theatre was pulled down.

5 Le Gallienne, p. 89. Sawday discusses the relationship of Pepys touching the body to the sovereign touch for scrofula and the paradoxical magic of the criminal corpse, *The Body Emblazoned*, pp. 77–8.

> Thence we went into a private room, where I perceive they prepare bodies, and there were the kidneys, ureters, etc., upon which he read to-day, and Dr. Scarborough, upon my desire and the company's, did show very clearly the manner of the disease of the stone and the cutting, and all other questions that I could think of.[6]

Pepys was especially interested in what he saw. Ten years earlier, in 1659, he had reluctantly had a bladder stone, reportedly the size of a tennis ball, removed by Thomas Hollyer (1609–90) a surgeon at St Thomas' and St Bartholomew's hospitals. Pepys was terrified of the operation, with good reason. The mortality rate was high – all four of the patients Hollyer operated on after Pepys died.[7]

Satisfied in his curiosity regarding the anatomical details of lithotomy, Pepys returned to the dinner table. There he and the medical men fell to discussing the use of silk and stiff ropes in hanging, pain and the greatest medical discovery of the age – the circulation of the blood. Pepys later wrote in his diary, 'that all the Doctors at table conclude, that there is no pain at all in hanging, for that it do stop the circulation of the blood, and so stops all sense and motion in an instant.'[8] Here we see Pepys juxtaposing the evidence presented by his feelings in seeing the body of someone hanged ('methought it an unpleasant sight') to the authoritative statements of the medical men ('there is no pain in hanging') to reach a state of uneasy acceptance of the knowledge of the medical community. The sight of the intact body had upset him; he was on much surer ground when it came to looking at the kidneys and ureters which lacked a personal identity.[9]

Pepys's experience at the Surgeons' Hall mirrored that of young Joseph Mede in the gardens of Cambridge University, who when confronted by a dead body 'asked what it meant?' Pepys had to be assured by the medical men gathered that his reaction to the body and the manner of the person's death was theoretically fallacious and emotionally incorrect. He followed William Harvey's advice in this matter:

> It behoves him, who ever is desirous to learn, to see any thing which is in question, if it be obvious to sense or sight, whether it be so or no, or else be bound to believe those that have made tryall, for by no other clearer or more evident certainty can he learn or be taught.[10]

Pepys accepted the vision of a community of medical practitioners who used experiential knowledge in certain ways both to define their studies and themselves.

6 *Idem.*

7 Pepys was number 31 in Hollyer's series for the year: numbers 32 through 35 all died. 'Pepys remained Hollyer's good friend and celebrated 26 March with a feast for the rest of his life.' Blandy, John P. and Lumley, John S. P., (eds) (2000), *The Royal College of Surgeons of England: 200 Years of History at the Millennium*, London: Blackwell Science Ltd., p. 8.

8 Le Galllienne, p. 89.

9 The bodies and the body parts were buried in a separate plot known as 'the anatomiser's ground' at St Olave's Parish Church. The Company paid for the burial. Murray and Hall, p. 53.

10 Harvey, William (1995), *The Anatomical Exercises: De Motu Cordis and De Circulatione Sanguinis in English Translation*, ed. Keynes, Geoffrey, New York: Dover Publications, p. 176.

These men were learned in anatomy and followed a Harveian programme of experiments that gave them a certain advantage. As anatomical skill could discipline the eyes, placing reason in control of the passions could discipline the mind. The head could be taught to rule the heart.

One person who self-consciously struggled with achieving dispassion was the physician, philosopher and prolific author Walter Charleton (1619–1707). He was the foremost proponent of Christian NeoEpicureanism in England and a leading member of both the Royal Society and the College of Physicians. Charleton was a friend of John Evelyn, Margaret Cavendish, Thomas Hobbes, William Harvey and John Wilkes.[11] He was also an acquaintance of Pepys:

> And at noon to dinner to the Popes head, where my Lord Brouncker (and his mistress dined) and Comissioner Pett, Dr. Charleton, and myself entertained with a venison pasty by Sir W. Warren. Here, very pretty discourse of Dr. Charleton concerning Nature's fashioning every creature's teeth according to the food she intends them. And that man's it is plain, was not for flesh, but for fruit. And that he can at any time tell the food of a beast unknown, by the teeth. My Lord Brouncker made one or two objections to it; that creatures find their food proper for their teeth, rather then that the teeth was fitted for the food. But the Doctor, I think, did well observe that creatures do naturally, and from the first, before they have experience to try, do love such a food rather then another. And that all children love fruit, and none brought to flesh but against their wills at first.[12]

Walter Charleton was interested in many subjects, from children's teeth and the origins of Stonehenge, to how to make the best wine. He wrote on the nature of the passions and the evils of atheism and produced a witty play that was performed on the London stage. Charleton was chosen to deliver the inaugural lectures at the new anatomy theatre at the College of Physicians in 1680. In an oft-repeated remark of the historian Charles Webster, Walter Charleton 'was very much the intellectual barometer of the age, and his numerous works are a valuable index to contemporary fashions.'[13] He was also the odd one out:

> Charleton also composed a not unimportant physiological textbook, *Oeconomia animalis* (1659), which appeared concurrently in a slightly abbreviated English form [as *Natural History of Nutrition, Life and Voluntary Motion*, London, 1659]. Such vernacular medical writings from academic physicians were somewhat unorthodox and philosophical in bias; they were composed for the benefit of a wider and possibly non-medical audience.[14]

---

11 Thompson, Helen (2002), 'Plotting Materialism: W. Charleton's The Ephesian Matron, E. Haywood's Fantomina, and Feminine Consistency', *Eighteenth Century Studies*, 35 (2), pp. 185–214. Rolleston, Humphrey (1940), 'Walter Charleton, D.M., F.R.C.P., F.R.S', *Bulletin of the History of Medicine*, (8), pp. 403–16.

12 (1985) *The Shorter Pepys*, selected and edited by Robert Latham, Berkeley: University of California Press, p. 645.

13 Webster, Charles (2002), *The Great Instauration, Science, Medicine and Reform, 1626–1660*, New York: Peter Lang, p. 278. For an excellent and succinct account of Charleton's life, see John Henry's entry in the *Oxford Dictionary of National Biography*, 2000, pp. 172–5.

14 Ibid., p. 282.

There is a thread, however, that weaves through all of Charleton's interests and that is his fascination with the passions and appetites as the bases for human actions. He read, wrote and dissected in order to draw conclusions about medicine, society and theology. As a result, studying Charleton reveals a great deal about the philosophical and emotional underpinnings of the medical community as it sought to survive the Civil War, the Interregnum and the restoration of the Stuarts.[15] In a world turned upside down where external control appeared impossible, many turned inwards to contemplate how to control their bodies and minds. Walter Charleton wrote and published about his struggles to achieve such control. He offered advice and mapped out a strategy. Charleton's works were widely read by famous men such as Robert Boyle, Isaac Newton and John Locke, but they also appealed to a wider community interested in medicine, philosophy and theology during a terrible era of political and spiritual turmoil.[16]

The intellectual barometer of his age

A son of a vicar from Shepton Mallet, Somerset, Charleton matriculated at Magdalen Hall, Oxford in 1635. Charles I gave him an MD upon mandate in 1643 and an appointment as a physician in ordinary. In 1653 the future Charles II would appoint him to a similar post, despite the king's exile in Europe. Oxford in the 1630s and 1640s was an exciting place to be if one had an interest in natural philosophy. Charleton was tutored by John Wilkins, later the founder of the Royal Society and the Bishop of Chester, and John Prideaux, Rector of Exeter College and later Vice Chancellor of the University and Bishop of Worcester. He became close friends with the diarist John Evelyn and the mathematician and first President of the Royal Society, William (later Viscount) Brouncker. The latter hosted the lunch at the Pope's Head where Pepys listened to Charleton and Brouncker debate the role of the teeth.

Charleton's connections did not end there. He attended William Harvey during the Oxford siege and later performed anatomical research on the nerves. He collaborated with Thomas Willis and Richard Lower as they investigated the structure of the nerves, brain and spleen and began to reorder anatomically the physical location of the passions. At Oxford he became acquainted with Charles Scarburgh along with the poet, Abraham Cowley and Henry Pierrepont, Marquis of Dorchester. Charleton's *Discourse concerning the Different Wits of Men* is said to have been consulted by John Locke.[17] Based on evidence from a letter that Lord Conway wrote to the royal

---

15 Jensen, H. James (ed.) (1996), *The Sensational Restoration*, Bloomington: Indiana University Press, p. 45.

16 Dear, Peter (1988), 'A Mechanical Microcosm: Bodily Passions, Good Manners, and Cartesian Mechanism,' in Lawrence, Christopher and Shapin, Steven, *Science Incarnate, Historical Embodiments of Natural Knowledge*, Chicago: University of Chicago Press, pp. 51–82, states 'the highest aim of Cartesian philosophy was proper behaviour', p. 63. The most complete biography of Descartes is Gaukroger, Stephen (1995), *Descartes: An Intellectual Biography*, Oxford: Clarendon Press.

17 Williamson, George (1989), *Seventeenth Century Contexts*, Chicago: University of Chicago Press, p. 166.

physician, Theodore de Mayerne (1573–1655) in September 1648, Charleton was also busy practising medicine.[18]

As a devout Royalist and high churchman, Charleton fled Oxford for London in 1649 and opened a fashionable medical practice in Russell Street, Covent Garden. He registered at the Royal College of Physicians upon his arrival and after a year-long struggle, was accepted as a candidate.[19] During the Interregnum he spent some time in the Netherlands and Paris where he met with the king in exile and became part of the 'Newcastle Circle' of Sir Kenelm Digby, Thomas Hobbes, George Ent and Margaret Cavendish. *The Immortality of the Human Soul, Demonstrated by the Light of Nature* (1657) is Charleton's most revealing work when it comes to describing the tribulations of being a Royalist physician in Commonwealth England. It consists of a dialogue about learning, civil war and morality between Athanasius (Charleton), Lucretius (Evelyn) and Isodicastes (Brouncker) as they stroll through the Luxembourg Gardens in Paris. First, Athanasius/Charleton gloomily sums up his life to Lucretius/Evelyn:

> ... from the time I first published that Physiology you mentioned, even to this very day, I have been embroil'd in as many troubles and distractions, as malice, persecution, and sharp adversity could accumulate upon me. I have been driven from my Country, House, Family, Books, Friends, and Acquaintance; and wholly depriv'd of all the chief endearments of life; insomuch that I am a perfect stranger to any such thing as comfort, but what I sometimes form to my self out of the assurance of my Innocence, and the hope of that compensation that is ordained for Patience in unjust sufferings.[20]

Charleton compares his life to one of a rudderless ship, where control is barely possible:

> In a word, Lucretius, (for as it sharpeneth the sense of my afflictions in my self, for me to recount them; for I know it cannot be, but very unpleasant to you, to hear the miserable adventures of your Friend for almost these two last years), I have been continually tos'd up and down by a Tempest of Calamity, which is yet so violent, that the dangers, which threaten me, seem to despise the prevention of that small skill I have in the use of my Compass: My Anchors are lost, my Vessell leaks, the Winds hurry it from land, and I hourly expect to sink down-right.[21]

Lucretius counsels his friend to avoid dwelling on his misfortunes as he already suffers from a melancholy disposition.[22] He introduces him to Isodicastes/Brouncker

18 Sharp, Lindsay (1973), 'Walter Charleton's Early Life 1620–1659, and Relationship to Natural Philosophy in Mid-Seventeenth Century England', *Annals of Science*, 30, p. 318.

19 *Idem*. Cook, Harold J. (1986), *The Decline of the Old Medical Regime in Stuart London*, Ithaca and London: Cornell University Press. Cook explains that 'Charleton's status as physician to Charles I raised questions for some members of the College. Perhaps his espousal of iatrochemistry and Epicureanism did too. Anyway, in 1655 Charleton was denied membership. He was finally elected to the Royal College of Physicians in 1676', p. 115.

20 Charleton, *The Immortality*, p. 11.

21 *Idem*.

22 Charleton, *The Immortality*, p. 13.

who asks for a report on 'the state of Learning in England'. And so begins the best-known part of Charleton's book, the description of the activities of *Solomons House* (the College of Physicians) and the *Benefactors of Learning* (the natural philosophers based in Oxford).[23] At the College they are carrying out comparative anatomy and 'Others there are, who daily investigate arguments to confirm and advance that incomparable invention of Doctor Harvey, the Circulation of the Blood.'[24]

In 1660 Charles II renewed Charleton's appointment as physician-in-ordinary. Ever the astute courtier, he quickly published *An Imperfect Pourtraicture of His Sacred Majesty Charles II* which cast the Merry Monarch in the role of a religious hermit. Charleton also dedicated his book to the king on the theory that Stonehenge was a meeting place for tribal chieftains of the Danes. To introduce *Chorea Gigantum* John Dryden composed the poem 'To my Honor'd Friend, Dr. Charleton, on his Learned and Useful Works'. Charleton's first book had also been on stones. *Spiritus Gorgonicus,* published in Leiden in 1650 was influenced by Van Helmont's *De Lithiasis* of 1644, but also included many of Charleton's own experiments and observations on urinary calculus.[25]

Charleton was a fellow of the Royal Society from its formation in 1660 and a fellow of the College of Physicians from 1676.[26] Active in both communities, Charleton carried out experiments with Robert Hooke at the Royal Society on grafting the skin from one dog to another and transplanting a spur to the head of a cock. Within the College he was appointed censor, senior censor, consilarius, president (three times) and also delivered the Harveian oration on three occasions. In 1677 he was appointed as the lecturer in anatomy at the College where his audience included his friend John Evelyn: 'I went to heare Dr. *Charletons* Lecture in the *Anatomie Theater* at the *Physitians Colledge*, upon the *heart*; and returned home.'[27] The same year Charleton published an illustrated work on comparative anatomy, *Exercitationes de Differentiis & Nominibus Animalium, Quibus accedunt Mantissa Anatomica*. It included an account with drawings of the dissection of the 'Toad-Fish or Fishing Frog'.

Charleton sank into poverty as he began to outlive his Royalist patients. In 1702 the surgeon James Yonge gave the following description of him, 'Charleton's age, hard study and misfortunes have somewhat soured him. He was now 82 years

23 Ibid., pp. 33–6. This description has been analysed by Webster, Charles (1967), 'The College of Physicians: "Solomon's House" in Commonwealth England', *Bulletin of the History of Medicine*, 41, pp. 393–412. Also see Andrew Cunningham (eds) (1996), 'The historical context of Wharton's work on the glands' in Freer, Stephen and Cunningham, Andrew *Thomas Wharton's Adenographia*, Oxford: Clarendon Press, pp. 27–52, especially pp.32–3. Cunningham notes that Charleton adopts a Baconian style when describing the College.

24 Charleton, *The Immortality*, p. 35.

25 Sharp, p. 321. Clericuzio, Antonio (2000), *Elements, Principles and Corpuscles: A Study of Atomism and Chemistry in the Seventeenth Century*, Boston and Dordrecht: Kluwer Academic Publishers, pp. 92–100.

26 Rolleston, p. 407.

27 De Beer, E.S, (ed.) (1955), *The Diary of John Evelyn*, Oxford: Clarendon Press, 4, p. 308.

old, yet strong and healthy, a genteel man in his behaviour, full of compliment ... .'[28] According to Anthony à Wood, Charleton divided his time between miserable lodgings in London and the Channel Island of Jersey, 'a learned and unhappy man ... yet too much given to romances.'[29] Wood had no reason to like him. John Aubrey reported that Charleton had delighted in collecting and publicising all the 'false Latins in Wood's book'.[30] In 1706 the College of Physicians, due to Charleton's destitution, appointed him Harveian Librarian with a stipend of £20. It was too little too late. A year later Walter Charleton died in abject poverty.

As can be seen, Charleton's writings were many and varied. The subjects reflected the effect of changing philosophical values on the medical community that, in turn, laid the groundwork for the emergence of a new type of learned practitioner – one able to realize the melding of knowledge, anatomical practices and theological values. During the Interregnum Charleton espoused one branch of the new mechanical philosophy, atomism. In particular, he admired the work of the professor of mathematics and astronomy at Paris, Pierre Gassendi (1592–1655). Charleton published a series of works on theology and atheism: *The Darkness of Atheism Dispelled by the Light of nature. A Physico-theological treatise* (1652), *Physiologia Epicuro-Gassendo-Charltonia: or a Fabrick of Science Natural upon the Hypothesis of Atoms* (1654), *The Immortality of the Human Soul, Demonstrated by the Light of Nature* (1657), and *Exercitationes Physico-anatomicae sive Oeconomia Animalis in medicina Hypothesibus Superstructurae* (1659).[31] Charleton's writings have not received a great deal of praise in the past three centuries. They are often described as translations, re-formulations or syntheses of other philosophers' works. Yet this is precisely what makes them so useful in showing what ideas caught the imagination of a community of medical men.[32]

Apparent in Charleton's writings was the importance of the new mechanical philosophy with its view of nature as ordered, regular and law-like. It was centred on an epistemology where gaining knowledge from both dispassionate observation and violent experiment was becoming the norm.[33] Rooted in the works of Epicurus,

28 *The Journal of James Yonge {1647–1721}, Plymouth Surgeon* (1963), F.N.L. Poynter (ed.), London: Longmans, p. 220.

29 Charleton, Walter, *Epicurus' Morals*, (1656), intro. Frederick Manning, London: Peter Davies, 1926, p. 17.

30 Balme, Maurice (2000), *Two Antiquaries: A Selection from the Correspondence of John Aubrey and Anthony Wood*, Durham: Durham Academic Press, p. 65.

31 On the slow emergence of Charleton's peculiar strain of atomism see Gelbart, Nina Rattner (November 1971), 'The Intellectual Development of Walter Charleton', *Ambix*, 18 (3), pp. 149–68.

32 This was recognized by Robert E. Kraus: 'In virtually all his pursuits and activities, Charleton was something less than brilliant ... his qualities of mind and activity were very much in line with those of many of his contemporaries with similar interests, education, and medical training.' See (1988), *Walter Charleton and The Natural History of Nutrition: Galenism in the Scientific Revolution*, M.A. Thesis, University of North Carolina, Chapel Hill, p.20.

33 There is a vast literature on early modern mechanical philosophy. The best study is still Brown, Theodore (1981), *The Mechanical Philosophy and the 'Animal Oeconomy'*, New

a Hellenistic Greek philosopher of the fourth and third centuries BC, and Lucretius, a Roman poet of the first century BC, the mechanical philosophy argued for the existence of tiny particles as the basis of all matter.

Controlling the body and mind

In the middle part of the seventeenth century Epicureanism enjoyed a revival in England. It was aided in large part by the efforts of Walter Charleton and John Evelyn, but also by the experience of the Civil War.[34] The NeoEpicureanism that resulted is best defined as a revival of Epicurus' temperate hedonism or, 'bread and water confer the highest possible pleasure' on 'hungry lips' (Diogenes Laertius 10.130–131):[35]

> Interregnum Royalists similarly expounded the Epicurean pleasure of temperance ... Walter Charleton, who had been Charles I's personal physician, claimed that a 'sober,' hungry man ate with 'more delight' than others.[36]

Evelyn cultivated gardens and Charleton mental calm in the face of disaster, both with Epicurus as their guide.[37]

Why was Epicurus so popular a role model? The Civil War and the ensuing religious chaos were major factors in attracting gentlemen to his doctrines, particularly those on the losing side in the 1640s and 1650s:

> The attraction of Epicureanism for Evelyn and other royalist sympathisers in the time of the Civil War lay above all in its emphasis on the principle of *ataraxia* – tranquillity achieved by avoiding extremes of passion and distress, not least by withdrawal from public affairs. The concept was interpreted by Walter Charleton in his *Epicurus' Morals* of 1656: 'Felicity doth consist ... in the stable kind of pleasure: and so can be no other, but the Indolency of Body, and Tranquillity of the Mind.' Consequently, 'A wise man is not to engage himself in the administration of Publick Affairs, unless some intervening Necessity call him thereunto'.[38]

While interest in the passions in seventeenth-century philosophy was part of the broader preoccupation in early modern Europe with the relation of knowledge of self

York: Arno Press.

34 Barbour, Reid (1998), *English Epicures and Stoics: Ancient Legacies in Early Stuart Culture*, Amherst: University of Massachusetts Press, p. 21. Barbour cites works by Margaret J. Osler and Robert Hugh Kargon, among others.

35 Scodel, Joshua (2002), *Excess and the Mean in Early Modern Literature*, Princeton: Princeton University Press, p. 259.

36 *Idem.*

37 See Carole and Alistair Small (1997), 'John Evelyn and the Garden of Epicurus', *Journal of the Warburg and Courtauld Institutes*, 60, pp. 194–214.

38 Small, p. 197.

to self-control, the situation in England left fewer options open for such interests.[39] As Walter Charleton said:

> Our late Warrs and Schisms, having almost wholly discouraged men from the study of theologie; and brought the Civil Law into contempt; the major part of young Schollers in our Universities addict themselves to Physick.[40]

It was safer to be a physician than a lawyer or a minister in times of political and religious turmoil. However studying the body and the passions rather than the soul, or God's laws, had its own dangers.

As an Epicurean atomist like Pierre Gassendi, Charleton was troubled by the atheism inherent in the theory that all was physical matter – for the ancients Democritus and Epicurus even the process of thought was purely a physical event. Charleton therefore strengthened Gassendi's argument that the soul was immaterial, making God both the Creator and director of all atomistic motion.[41] The soul, however, continued to act in a mechanistic way. In Charleton's and many others' view the English Civil War had given rise to 'swarms of Atheisticall Monsters'. In *The Darkness of Atheism dispelled by the Light of Nature* (1652) Charleton attempted to support traditional religion with natural philosophy, particularly the immortality and immateriality of the soul and the existence of God the Creator.[42] Mechanics and mathematical quantification, while explaining a great deal, fall short of being a sufficient system. God and his generously bestowed spirits and faculties must be included too, and Charleton laments that Epicurus could have thought otherwise. It is truly astonishing, he says of Epicurus, that 'so much of the Scholar, and so much of the Fool could have met ... in one and the same brain.'[43]

As Margaret Osler has expertly shown, Charleton, like Descartes, based his philosophy of nature on theological foundations.[44] Descartes's works first entered

---

39 See Scodel. Also Dear, 'A Mechanical Microcosm: Bodily Passions, Good Manners, and Cartesian Mechanism'.

40 Gascoigne, John (1990), 'A reappraisal of the role of the universities in the Scientific Revolution', *Reappraisals of the Scientific Revolution*, Lindberg, David C. and Westman, Robert S. (eds), Cambridge: Cambridge University Press, pp. 207–60, see p. 242. In *The Immortality of the Human Soul*, Charleton states, 'The universities have a great share in all these ill ways by their first bringing up and breeding their young student(s). For they have left the old and sound Aristotle learning, and spend all their time in the new-fangles fripperies of Cartes, Gassendus, Boyle, Hobbs and Regius, etc.' p. 311.

41 'Charleton's defense of Epicurus's errors is that the truth of the immortality of the sol and the illegality of suicide is difficult to discover without revelation, and that Epicurus did not have this advantage.' Kroll, Richard W. F. (1991), *The Material Word: Literate Culture in the Restoration and the Early Eighteenth Century*, Baltimore: The Johns Hopkins University Press, p. 56.

42 Charleton, Walter (1654), *Physiologia, Epicuro-Gassendo-Charltonia: Or a Fabrick of Science Natural upon the Hypothesis of Atoms*, p. xix.

43 Quoted in Gelbart, p.162. It comes from Charleton's (1652), *The Darkness of Atheism Dispelled by the Light of Nature, A Physico-Theologicall Treatise*, London, p. 60.

44 Osler, Margaret J. (1979), 'Descartes and Charleton on Nature and God', *Journal of the History of Ideas*, 40 (3), pp. 445–56, quotation from p. 452.

England in 1644 as translations into Latin. In 1650 they were published anonymously in London as *The Passions of the Soule, in three bookes*. Descartes's ideas certainly influenced Charleton, Willis, Lower and others in the Oxford community who contemplated the physical location and operation of the passions within the body. In turn they affected the ways in which medical men regarded their own bodies and those of their patients.[45]

Descartes obtained his anatomical knowledge first-hand in the yards of butchers, and his work was therefore appealing to admirers of Harvey's bloody endeavours. Like other devout dissectors Descartes found it necessary both to defend and to praise his inclinations. In Amsterdam he often watched the slaughtering of cattle and then had the parts that he wanted to dissect carried to his lodgings. This appears to have become well known among the residents of Amsterdam, along with his journeys into the countryside to watch pigs being killed. Descartes apparently felt he had to defend his interests and expressed gratitude for the understanding of Mersenne in a letter he wrote to the Minim friar in 1639:

> Mais comme vous m'écrivez, ce n'est pas un crime d'être curieux de l'anatomie; et j'ai été en hiver à Amsterdam, que j'allais quasi tous les jours en la maison d'un boucher, pour lui voir tuer des bêtes, et faisais apporter de là en mon logis les parties que je voulais anatomiser plus a loisir; ce que j'ai encore fait plusiers fois en tous les lieux où j'ai été, et je ne crois pas qu'aucun homme d'esprit m'en puisse blâmer.[46]

Pain was something all humans wrestled with, physicians and surgeons in particular. Descartes famously gave a purely mechanical explanation of pain – a foot which comes into contact with fire is involuntarily withdrawn because the moving particles of fire cause the skin to move. A thin thread is then pulled which opens a valve in the brain and animal spirits are then transmitted through the hollow canals of nerves to the muscles. This causes the foot to pull back from the fire:

> If the filaments that compose the marrow of these nerves are pulled with force enough to be broken and thus are separated from the part to which they were joined, so that the

45 Père Marin Mersenne (1588–1654) was a Minim friar, 'who made himself the centre of an extensive network of natural philosophers'. Henry, John (1992), 'The Scientific Revolution in England', in *The Scientific Revolution in National Context*, Porter, Roy and Teich, Mikuláš (eds), Cambridge and New York: Cambridge University Press, pp. 178–209.

Descartes stated he had been dissecting like this for 11 years in a letter to Mersenne on 20 February 1639.

46 Lindeboom, Dr G.A. (1979), *Descartes and Medicine*, Amsterdam: Rodolphi Press, p. 37. 'But as you wrote, it isn't a crime to be curious about anatomy; and when I have been in Amsterdam during winter, I went nearly everyday to a butcher's yard to witness the slaughter, and caused to be brought to my lodgings the parts of the beasts I wanted to dissect at greater leisure; and I have often done this in other places where I stayed, and I don't believe that any honourable man should blame me for such activities.' Jonathon Sawday notes that Rembrandt also haunted abattoirs and even speculates that he might have met Descartes in *The Body Emblazoned,* pp. 161–3.

structure of the whole machine is somewhat less intact, the movement they then cause in the brain will cause the soul ... to experience a feeling of *pain*.[47]

The passions, therefore, have a direct relation to muscular motion via the animal spirits passing through the nerves. The direction and flow of the animal spirits from the brain to the muscles depended to a large extent upon the micro-structure of the spirits themselves, which in turn was affected by the disposition of specific organs and the impressions of external objects upon the senses.[48]

In the aforementioned *The Passions of the Soule* (1650), Descartes's discussion of the relation of pain to particular passions included a section titled 'pitty'. Pity was described as a sort of sadness mingled with love or goodwill towards those afflicted. Those who were weak and prone to fancies suffered the most from pity, although the most generous men were also susceptible to this passion, albeit with significant differences:

(B)ut the Sadness of this (generous men's) Pitty is not bitter, and like that which tragicall actions personated on the stage cause, is more in the exteriours and the senses, than the interiours of the Soul, which in the mean is satisfied to think she hath done her duty, in that she hath a fellow feeling with the afflicted; and there is this difference in it, that wheras the vulgar pitty those who complain, because they think the ills they suffer are very grievous, the principall object of great mens Pitty is the weaknesse of those that they see complain; because they esteem not any accident that may befall to be no great an evill, as is the Baseness of those who cannot suffer constantly; and though they hate the vices, yet they hate not those they see subject to them: they only Pitty them.[49]

Cartesian philosophy fitted well with the desires of some English medical men to discipline their emotions when dissecting, vivisecting or contemplating their own bodies. To achieve absolute dominion of the passions a rational mind required extensive training in filtering and even ignoring the signals of the body. Descartes provided help in defining the body as a machine in the *Meditations on First Philosophy* (1641). The soul was pure *res cogitans* – conscious and incorporeal, while the body was *res extensa* – unconscious and brutish material.[50] In one of the most famous passages from *Meditations*, Descartes bluntly stated that the 'life' of the body was solely a mechanical function:

[W]e may judge that the body of a living man differs from the that of a dead man just as does a watch or other automaton, when it is wound up and contains in itself the corporeal

47 Descartes, René (1972), *Treatise of Man*, trans. Thomas Steele Hall, Cambrdige, MA: Harvard University Press, 1972, p. 37.

48 Wright, John P. (1990), 'Hysteria and Mechanical Man', in Yolton, John W. (ed.), *Philosophy, Religion, and Science in the Seventeenth and Eighteenth Centuries*, Rochester: University of Rochester Press, pp. 233–47, quotation from p. 240. Also see Niebyl, Peter H. (1971), 'The Non Naturals': A Note on the Origins and Fate of a Doctrine and a Phrase', *Bulletin of the History of Medicine*, 45, pp. 486–92.

49 Descartes René, (1650) *The Passions of the Soule,* London, p.153.

50 Bordo, Susan R. (1987), *The Flight To Objectivity: Essays On Cartesianism & Culture*, New York: State University of New York Press, p. 93.

> principle of these movements for which it is designated along with all that is requisite for its action, from the same watch or other machine when it is broken and when the principle of its movement ceases to act.[51]

In contrast to Descartes, Charleton stressed God's exercise of free will resulting in a very different attitude towards the laws of nature and human knowledge. Empirical methods had to be employed to find out about them. As Margaret Osler notes, Charleton's 'theory of knowledge emphasizes observation and experience, without being narrowly empiricist.'[52] The senses were not reliable when it came to finding out about the material world – they could only approximate truth. Charleton returned again and again to this problem of the relation of reason to the passions. How could the rational soul and the sensitive soul be brought into harmony? How could we learn to curb our most violent sensual responses and acquire the Epicurean virtue of tranquillity of mind or dispassion? In particular, what did such goals mean in terms of being part of an emotional community of medical men? In attempting this great project Charleton found some comfort in William Harvey's work on blood. The *Two Discourses: I. Concerning the Different Wits of Men. II. Of the Mysterie of Vintners* (1669), included a discussion of the purity of wits, wine and blood:

> Our perspicacious Countryman Dr. *Harvey*, somewhere in his Book of the *Generation of Animals*, affirms it to be no small advantage to the Brain, that Students and contemplative Men preserve their mass of Blood pure and uncorrupt.[53]

As a very contemplative natural philosopher, Charleton was therefore blessed with a particularly rational brain.

The ideal medical man

Examining a diverse selection of Charleton's works over several decades gives us an opportunity to take a deeper look at the ideas and activities of this 'intellectual barometer'. The three works chosen are first, *The Ephesian Matron* (1659), a witty story incorporating much of his anatomical and religious interests, second,

51 Ibid., p. 94.

52 Osler, 'Descartes and Charleton', p. 454.

53 Charleton, Walter (1669), *Two Discourses. I. Concerning the Different Wits of Men: II. Of the Mysterie of Vintners*, London, p. 50.

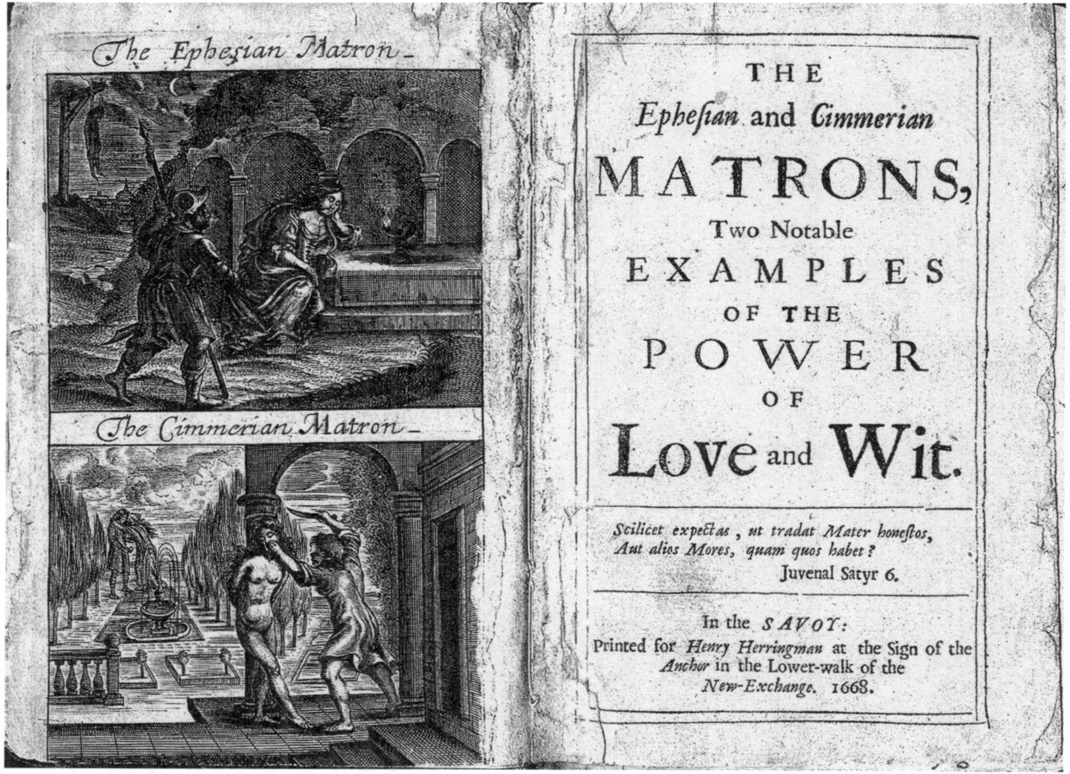

Figure 2.1 **Title page of Walter Charleton's *The Ephesian and Cimmerian Matrons*, London, 1668. Courtesy of the US National Library of Medicine.**

the *Natural History of the Passions* (1674),[54] where Charleton researched 'the most powerfull Remedies against ... Excesses of the passions'[55] and third, *Enquiries Into Human Nature in VI Anatomic Praelections in the new Theatre of the Royal Colledge of Physicians in London,* a lengthy address followed by lectures on nutrition and the heart, given in 1680.[56]

Charleton composed all these works as medico-philosophical treatises to achieve a common end. In the story he dissects the passions of the Ephesian Matron and her lover; in his book on the history of the passions, he dissects himself; and in the lectures at the College's new theatre, he dissects the human body and the act of anatomizing itself. Charleton saw medical knowledge, specifically anatomical knowledge, as essential to all these projects.

In 1659 Charleton published *The Ephesian Matron*, a reinterpretation of the ancient story of 'The Widow of Ephesus', found in the Stoic Gaius Petronius' *The Satyricon*.[57]

The plot as rewritten by Charleton revealed much about his interest in religion and the passions and his belief that as an anatomist he was in a unique position to reveal not only the workings of the body but also of the mind:

> I say, that neither is the knowledge of the Passions to be acquir'd without frequenting the Scholes of Anatomists. For the Passions seem to be in general, only certaine Commotions of the Spirits and bloud, begun in the seat of the Imagination, propagated through the Pathetic nerves to the heart, and thence transmitted up again to the brain.[58]

54 This has been sometimes taken in the past to be a translation of Jean-François Senault's *De l'usage des passions*, Paris, 1641, but it is not. Senault was translated by Henry Earl of Monmouth in 1649 as *The Uses of the Passions, Written in French by J.F. Senault*, with a second edition in 1671. See Hunter, Richard A. and Cuttler, Emily (January 1958), 'Walter Charleton's Natural History of the Passions (1674) and J.F. Senault's The Use of Passions (1649): A Case of Mistaken Identity', *Journal of the History of Medicine*, pp. 87–92. For a lucid discussion of the history of the story Charleton adapted, see, Carleton, Samuel (1973), *Pétrone Démoralisé: 'The Ephesian Matron' of John Ogilby*, dissertation, the University of Texas at Austin.

55 Thorpe, Clarence DeWitt (1940), *The Aesthetic Theory of Thomas Hobbes*, University of Michigan Press, p. 181.

56 According to Rolleston, this was an extensive revision and at least the seventh edition of the *Natural History of nutrition, life, and voluntary motion. Containing all the new discoveries of anatomists and most probable opinions of physicians concerning the oeconomie of human nature*. The six lectures concerned nutrition, the stomach, the ventricle, life, fevers and voluntary motion. The Dedication was new as was the Epistle and parts of the Epilogue in the 1659 edition.

57 There were other editions in 1658, 1659 and 1668. It was translated into Latin in 1665 by Bartholomew Harris. The 1658 and 1668 editions were published with *The Cimmerian Matron* by P.M. Gent. See the introduction to Charleton, Walter (1975), *The Ephesian Matron* (1668), by Guibbory, Achsah Los Angeles: William Andrews Clark Memorial Library. All quotations are from the 1668 Gent edition.

58 Charleton, *The Ephesian Matron*, Preface, p. 11.

Petronius' story had long been popular in England and on the Continent. A newly widowed young woman is found mourning at her husband's tomb by a soldier who has entered the vault to seek shelter for the night. He revives the trembling and half-starved woman with wine and food. This leads to them being overcome with sexual desire and they make love. When the heat of passion has subsided, the couple find that the corpse of a thief which the soldier was to guard has been stolen. In order to protect him from punishment the young widow substitutes her husband's corpse for that of the thief.

Charleton embroidered the story with philosophical passages and used his anatomical and theological knowledge to educate his audience on love, lust and survival.[59] He began his tale with a scene that would have been very familiar to him, and perhaps even hinted at the difficulty the College of Physicians had in wresting bodies for dissection away from family and friends of the hanged:

> On the very same day her Husband's funeral rites were solemnized ... there was a notorious malefactor executed, and his body left upon the Gibbet; the better to strike terror into others ... and lest any of the Villain's relations or confederates, should take down the mangled Carcass, and convey it away to burial privily in the night ... a guard of Soldiers [was] confined to watch it ... .[60]

Charleton added several scenes to the story, including a long digression on the passion of love. He stated that we choose our partners, much as we choose food and drink, in order to satiate our appetites. The choice has little to do with any moral or religious qualities the person may have. In the story, the widow is revived with food and drink and she quickly moves from suicidal thoughts to ones of perpetual life through getting pregnant by the soldier and producing children. Charleton does not fully adopt the view of his friend Thomas Hobbes that self-preservation is blameless liberty and how we sort good from evil. Instead he adopts an ironic and dispassionate tone and changes Petronius' story to highlight the violence of womanly passion, 'for her Humour you will find her in all things a perfect Woman, a little subject to changes ... leaping at once out of a Charnel-house into a Nuptial-bed.'[61]

Charleton was deeply interested in nutrition and had also published on vintners; he highlights his special knowledge of the interaction of the guts and wine with anatomical details and a pithy wit. The soldier revives the matron with wine but she swoons once more and this time he:

---

59 'The changes are primarily in the explanations of the characters' motivations, and the inclusion of details such as the soldier's passions, the details of the mutilation of the late husband's body, and the passages purportedly from Chaucer.' *The Sensational Restoration,* p. 42.

60 Charleton, *The Ephesian Matron*, p. 6.

61 *Idem*. See Charleton, Walter (1669), *The Mysterie of Vintners: Or A Brief Discourse concerning the various Sicknesses of WINES, and their respective Remedies, at this Day commonly used,* London. This was originally delivered as a lecture to the Royal Society at Gresham College on 26 November 1662.

> ... holds up her head with one hand, while with the other he drencheth her with a round dose of the remaining liquor ... and she became the most affable, compleasant, and chearfull creature in the world, indeed as if a new Soul had been infused into her.[62]

Charleton also manages to make sideswipes at contemporary social mores such as the so-called 'Modern Platoniques'. These profess to love purely but in fact hypocritically conceal their true sexual natures. Unlike in ancient times, these relationships exist between the different sexes, 'in the scorching years of life',[63] with the lovers married to others. Such love is 'Cousin German'[64] to the lust of the Ephesian Matron and her soldier.[65] Charleton did not have far to look for an example of platonic love. As Frances Harris has revealed in *Transformation of Love*, Charleton's friend, the married John Evelyn, made no secret of his feelings for the young Margaret Godolphin before and after her marriage.[66]

Petronius had the soldier wooing the distraught young woman; Charleton describes the seduction of the soldier by the woman and intercourse taking place on top of her husband's coffin. The scene is described with a mixture of crude and sly wit:

> I perceive, he hath not yet exhausted all his Ammunition, and that ... he is arming himself for a second encounter ... Let us, therefore, reasonably divert our yet innocent Eyes, and leave these her new votaries quietly to finish those *Cytherean* Rites they are going about: especially since their Zeal is so fervent, as not to scruple at the nicety of making the Dead Husband's Coffin, the Altar, whereon to kindle and exhale the incense they have brought.[67]

As with the widow, Charleton also invests the soldier with violent passions not found in Petronius. On finding the thief's corpse missing and knowing that the penalty for his failure to guard it will be his own execution, he turns on the woman and asks, 'What damned Spirit was it that conducted me into this Charnel-house, and made me

62 Ibid., p. 22.

63 Ibid., p. 66.

64 Ibid., p. 68.

65 George Williamson briefly discusses *The Ephesian Matron* as an attack on the hypocrisy of the cult of Platonic Love which had been rife in the court of Charles I and had its adherents after the Restoration. See *Seventeenth Century Contexts*, pp.289–93. Charleton had married in 1650 but we do not even know what his wife's first name was. Her father was the rector, Bartholomew Parsons *c.*1574–1642 and Charleton performed an autopsy on him in January 1671 in Wiltshire. There were no children. In his collection of *Epicurus' Morals*, London, of 1656 (reprinted 1670) Charleton objected to marriage as it could lead to 'Consumption of strength, decay of Industry, unfitness for business and labour, neglect of Domestick Prudence, impairment of Estate, Mortgages, and Forfeitures, ruine of reputation and Fame.' p. 73. One suspects he and his wife were not close.

66 Harris, Frances (2003), *Transformation of Love: The Friendship of John Evelyn and Margaret Godolphin*, Oxford: Oxford University Press.

67 Charleton, *Ephesian Matron*, p. 35.

quit my duty? ... Would I had fallen into a den of Lyons and Tygers, when I lighted upon this Woman here.'[68]

Quickly the woman devises an anatomically sound and dispassionate plan to substitute the body of her husband for the missing corpse of the thief. She points out that:

> ... it is but Charity to use the reliques of the Dead, in case of necessity, to preserve the Living: why should not I dispense with the Formality of posthume Respects to the putrifying Corps of my deceased Husband ... Come, therefore, my Dear, and let us take my Husbands body out of his Coffin and place it upon the Gibbet, in the room of the Malefactor, which you say has been stolen away.[69]

How the passion of lust has changed the Ephesian Matron from a weeping widow to the soldier's mistress is represented by Charleton in the violence of the acts she now proposes to protect her new love:

> Death (you know) doth so change & disfigure the Countenance, as to disguise it from the knowledge of even the most familiar Acquaintance. Who then can distinguish this his naked body from the other, besides, we will besmear his face with blood and dirt, and rather than fail in any part of resemblance, break his Arms and Legs, and make the same wounds in him, the Executioner did in the Rogue's ... [70]

The soldier follows her instructions and the tale ends with them in his lodgings happily planning their future together.

This theme of the ways in which the excesses of passion can drive us to act against all reason was one that Charleton returned to repeatedly. Emulating Epicurus, he devoted time to studying his emotional responses to pain and suffering. The *Natural History of the Passions* (1674) began with a reference to the ten weeks of solitary contemplation Charleton had spent in the countryside arranging his 'Philosophical papers ... wherein among other things, I had formerly, out of the best Authors, made certain *Collections* concerning the divine art of acquiring constant *Tranquillity* of Mind, by *Wisedom* or the right use of Reason.'[71] Charleton chose to seclude himself because he was suffering from discontent and wished to find the most effectual remedies. Like a good physician he sought to heal himself through recognizing that the 'attaining of internal serenity consisted principally in directing our desires aright'[72] towards things that we know to be good. The question then became: how do we know if a thing is good? Charleton digested his collections and private sentiments and constructed an order or method to describe the passions:

> I put them also into a dress of *Language* so plain and familiar, as may alone evince, my design was to write of this Argument, neither as an Orator, nor as a Moral Philosopher,

68 Ibid., p. 72.

69 Ibid., p. 78.

70 *Idem.*

71 Charleton, Walter (1674), *Natural History of the Passions*, London, the Epistle Prefatory, p. 1.

72 Ibid., p. 4.

> but only as a *Natural* one conversant in *Pathology*, and that too more for his own private satisfaction, than the instruction of others. And thus have I succinctly acquainted you with the *Occasion*, *Subject*, *Scope* and *Stile* of the Treatise that accompanieth this Epistle.[73]

Besides Epicurus and Hobbes, Charleton looked to Descartes as a source. He was particularly scathing, however, of Descartes's description of the pineal gland as the site of the rational soul:

> ... that had this excellent Man, *Monsieur des Cartes* been but half as conversant in Anatomy, as he seems to have been in Geometry, doubtles [sic] he would never have lodged so noble a guest as the Rational Soul in so incommodious a closet of the brain, as the *Glandula Pincalis* is; the *use* whereof hath been demonstrated to be no other but to receive into is spongy cavities, from two little nerves; a certain serous Excrement ... .[74]

Furthermore, Charleton states he has seen the *Glandule* and knows it is not flexible but fixed. It would not move even if the 'greatest Hurricano (sic) of spirits imaginable'[75] excited it.

Descartes was not the only one who could err. How skillful an anatomist Charleton actually was is debatable. On 22 October 1664, with the support of the Royal Society, Charleton publicly dissected a body at Gresham College. Five days later Henry Oldenburg wrote to Robert Boyle with exciting news, 'Dr. Charleton affirmed ... YT ye veines on ye right and left side of ye heart were transposed, so YT ye vena arteries was where the arteria venosa useth to be and vicissim.'[76] In other words the blood structure of the chest was reversed. Moreover, Dr Charles Scarburgh had dissected a body at Gresham College the very same day and found it lacked a 'musculus pectoralis'.[77] Charleton told Scarburgh of the transposed vessels and he was keen to disinter parts of the two dissected corpses in order to examine the heart for the first time and to see his own discovery again. This was done and much embarrassment ensued. On 3 November 1664 Oldenburg again wrote to Boyle:

> Dr. Charleton being calld to an account of his last dissection, and particularly pressed concerning ye Transposition, wch I mentioned to you in my former from his own mouth in ye presence of others, who heard him as well, as I, alledge Dr Ent for a witnesse of his assertion, was obliged at our yesterday's assembly at Gresham to yield, YT he was mistaken; both Dr Ent, who was wth us, and Dr Scarborough, having, upon ye unburying of ye heart, and a strict search and examination, found no such transposition; wch discovery of ye Drs error, spread by his very positive affirmations (wch made me wthout scruple deliver it also to you) addeth but very little to his credit. In ye meane time, ye other Anatomicall Observation concerning ye defect of ye Pectorall muscle is confirmed, Dr Ent himselfe, upon my particular inquiry asserting it with all confidence, and YT ye person, whilst alive, had not appeared defective in his motions.[78]

---

73 Ibid., p. 7.

74 Ibid., p. 16.

75 Ibid., p. 17.

76 Henry Oldenburg (*d.*1677) was the Secretary of the Royal Society.

77 *The Correspondence of Henry Oldenburg* (1966), trans. and ed. Hall, A. Rupert and Hall, Marie Boas, Madison: University of Wisconsin Press, 2, p. 273.

78 Ibid., 2, p. 280–81.

This anatomical duel tells us of the rivalry among the emotional community of the leading physicians and natural philosophers in London. By the 1660s anatomical expertise was something the heirs of William Harvey prided themselves in having – it was essentially an English virtue. Charleton had even attended Harvey at Oxford in the 1640s and aided the great Thomas Willis in his dissections and vivisections. Scarburgh and George Ent were close friends of Harvey. Oldenburg makes sure that Boyle knows he was not the only one who heard Charleton's claim – Ent was there too.

Scarburgh and Ent publicly examined the heart in front of members of the Royal Society and no doubt in front of members of the College of Physicians as well. This must have been humiliating for Charleton, especially as they found no anomaly to marvel at in his dissection except Charleton's incompetence. He had even failed in dissecting the most Harveian of organs – the heart. Meanwhile Scarburgh was praised as the discoverer of the truth, not only for his discovery of the lack of a pectoral muscle but because he also had discovered Charleton's ineptitude.

This one anecdote is not enough to condemn Charleton's anatomical skills. He certainly professed to have them and his explanation of the passions in *The Natural History* was based on his knowledge of dissecting and seeing the interiors of bodies. For example, sorrow is partly manifested by sighing. Sighing, in turn, is caused by the lungs being almost empty of blood:

> ... when some sudden imagination of *Hope* or comfort opens the sluice of the *Arteria Venosa* in the lungs, which sorrow had lately contracted. For, then that little blood that remained in the lungs, in a moment passing down through that pipe into the left ventricle of the heart; the ambient aire instantly rusheth by the mouth into the lungs, to replenish that place the blood had left free: and this *great and quick repletion of the lungs with aire*, is what we call *Sighing*.[79]

Weeping was caused by the lungs being stuffed and distended with blood – it was the opposite of sighing. In this context the Ephesian matron and her soldier-lover were a system of sluice gates and dykes through which the passions rushed. Heavily influenced by Thomas Hobbes's *Human Nature* (1650), Charlton concluded his *Natural History* with the passions being cast as false deceivers suggesting 'exorbitant desires' to us, 'upon which all the *Good* and *Evil* incident to us in this life seems to depend.'[80]

In 1676 Thomas Shadwell (1640–92) satirized natural philosophers like Charleton who lay around for weeks in the countryside contemplating their navels.[81] In his play *The Virtuoso*, however, he supported Charleton's view that everyone behaves according to their passions and appetites. As in *The Ephesian Matron* the

79 Charleton, *Natural History*, p. 158.

80 Ibid., p. 3.

81 On the image of the solitary philosopher see Shapin, Steven (1990), 'The Mind Is Its Own Place: Science and Solitude in Seventeenth-Century England', *Science in Context*, 4 (1), pp. 191–218. Shapin notes that solitude was widely regarded as a practical necessity for the scholar but if a gentleman retired from his public 'calling', it was seen as 'licenses to idleness, trivial pursuits and debauch'. p. 199.

strongest motive for action in *The Virtuoso* was sexual and the plot owed something to Epicurus. *The Virtuoso* was even dedicated to William Cavendish, Duke of Newcastle, (1592–1676) husband of Charleton's friend, Margaret Cavendish.

The protagonist of *The Virtuoso* has no feelings for others, his passions are reserved for himself and his experiments. Often seen as partly a satire on the Royal Society, and specifically on Robert Hooke, some scenes in *The Virtuoso* also poke fun at the dispassionate philosopher who lolls about achieving nothing of use. Perhaps, this shows how far Neo-Epicureanism had penetrated popular culture.

Act 2, Scene 2 finds Sir Nicholas Gimcrack, the Virtuoso, learning to swim like a frog on the table. He is attended by Longvil and Bruce, 'two gentlemen of wit and sense' and Sir Formal Trifle, 'a florid coxcomb':

> SIR NICH. Nay, I doubt not, sir, in a very little time to become amphibious; a man, by art, may appropriate any element to himself. You know a great many *virtuoso's* that can fly ...
> LONGV. Have you ever tri'd in the water, sir?
> SIR NIC. No, sir; but I swim most exquisitely on land.
> BRUCE. Do you intend to practise in the water, sir?
> SIR NIC. Never, sir; I hate the water, I never come upon the water, sir.
> LONG. Then there will be no use of swimming.
> SIR NIC. I content myself with the speculative part of swimming, I care not for the practice. I seldom bring anything to use, 'tis not my way, knowledge is my ultimate end.
> BRUCE. You have reason, sir; knowledge is like virtue, its own reward.
> SIR FORM. To study for use is base and mercenary, below the serene and quiet temper of a sedate philosopher.[82]

Twenty-one years after the publication of *The Ephesian Matron* and six years after *The Natural History of the Passions*, Charleton gave six inaugural lectures in anatomy at the new anatomy theatre at the College of Physicians in Warwick Lane, which was designed by Robert Hooke. He began the first lecture in anatomy ever carried out at the new theatre with a lengthy address to the College detailing the illustrious history of anatomy. Charleton followed it with *Enquiries Into Human Nature in IV Anatomic Praelections.* The lectures were accompanied by dissections.

In his address, Charleton, not surprisingly, first drew attention to the universal benefits for mankind of having such a theatre, namely the piety towards God it would inspire:

> Evident it is then, that Your *Theatre* may be properly enough call'd, a *Temple* of *Natural Theology*, where the *Perfections* of God are studied in the Works of His hands, and his *Praises* celebrated with Understanding. *Deum enim colit, qui novit.*[83]

While the theatre was a temple designed for worship of the art of anatomy, the subject of the art, the cadaver, was but some soulless machine. In fact Charleton constantly referred to the human body as an *automaton*:

---

82 Jensen, *The Sensational Restoration*, p. 395.

83 Charleton, Walter (1680), *Enquiries Into Human Nature,* the Epistle Dedicatory, p. 1.

My SUBJECT *is, the most abstruse* Oeconomy *of Nature in the body of Man; a System of innumerable smaller* Machines *or Engines, by infinite Wisdom fram'd and compacted into one most beautiful, greater* Automaton: *all whose parts are among themselves different in their sensibilities ... yet all ordain'd and adjusted to one common End, namely, to compose a Living* Ergasterium *or Work-house, in which a* Reasonable *and* Immortal Soul *may ... exercise all her divine Faculties.*[84]

Mechanist analogies have long histories – Aristotle compared the motions of organisms to that of automata. Galen compared the respiratory system to mechanical bellows arrangement.[85] Charleton was drawing upon the tradition in his statement:

My PROVINCE *is, the* Anatomic Administration *of these ruines of a Man*, i.e. *to take asunder some few at least of the various* Organs *of this Master-piece of the Creation, so that we may explore their several conduit-pipes, their springs, movements, actions, communications, offices, in fine, their whole* Mechanism ...[86]

For Charleton the body while alive was, unless brought under control by the exercise of reason, subject to its passions. Once dead the body was a machine-corpse that could be admired, manipulated and, crucially, be of anatomical and religious service. As the Ephesian matron dryly commented, 'it is but Charity to use the reliques of the dead.' The passions were never far from Charleton's mind. Did his audience perhaps expect the physician who had dedicated his life to understanding the war between reason and emotion to lecture on his passion?

According to Charleton the passions arose from the blood:

Therefore whosoever would duly enquire into their nature ... will soon find himself under a necessity to begin at Anatomy, thence to learn the course of the bloud, the origin and productions of the nerves, the fabric of the heart with its pulses ... Otherwise, how highly soever he might think of his own speculations, he would hardly be able clearly to solve any one of the Phaenomena *of this or that particular Passion; for instance, whence it is, that* Blushing *is the proper sign of* Shame, Paleness *the Character of suddain* Fear, Sadness *the inseparable concomitant of* Hate, *& sic de cœteris. In a word, he would as soon be at a loss in tracing the intricate Labyrinth of Human Affections, as a blind man that should undertake to give the Chorography of a whole Countrey, meerly from a relation of some memorable action done in some part of it.*[87]

Charleton also addressed physiognomy in *The Ephesian Matron*, where he carefully described the changes in the title character's skin colour, the tenor of her voice, her sparkling eyes after being plied with wine by the soldier. She 'appears now to have so little of the sorrowful Widow in her, that if I might have the liberty Physiognomists take, of divining by outward signes, I should take her for the most pleased and happy

84 Ibid., Preface, p. 1.

85 Hall, Thomas S. (1969), *The History of General Physiology*, Chicago: University of Chicago Press, 1, p. 222.

86 Charleton, *Enquiries*, Preface, p. 2.

87 Ibid., Preface, p. 4.

Bride in the world.'[88] Charleton's explanation for her change was based on close anatomical observation and physiological knowledge:

> A temperate and Balmy Sweat, extilling from the pores of her snow-white skin, helps to increase the kindly warmth of it, arising, doubtless, from a great agitation of her spirits within, and an effusion of them upon the outward parts … .'[89]

In other words, she was glowing.[90]

Harvey had mapped out the labyrinth of the body for his students; Charleton strove to do the same for the passions. It was the key to self-knowledge and self-control. Following his passage on the necessity to practise anatomy in order to understand the foundations of the passions, Charleton turned the argument around and made an eloquent case for dissection affecting the passions of the anatomist:

> *Nor should I believe such a man half so likely to temper and compose the tumults of his inordinate* Passions, *as a skilful* Anatomist, *who understands, by what impressions they are occasion'd, upon what parts of the brain those impressions are made, what sympathy and confederation* Nature *has instituted between those parts and the* Cardiac *nerves, how those nerves divided into innumerable fibres contract the ventricles of the heart, and how that* Contraction, *according to the various degrees of its force and velocity, necessarily impells the blood more or less copiously and violently through the arteries into the parts most concern'd in the* Passion *at that time most urgent.* [91]

Anatomical knowledge gave Charleton and his audience a strategy for managing their wilful bodies. They were privileged because they knew how their bodies worked from examining the bodies of others. They could thus cultivate reason:

> *For, certainly, he that hath the advantage to understand all these things, is better instructed to appease the impetuous Commotions at any time rais'd within his breast, by reducing the rebellious appetites of his inferior Faculties to obedience to the contremands of his Superior or Reason; in which one thing the summ of all* Moral Philosophy *consists, and which advanced into a* Habit, *becomes* Virtue *itself.*[92]

Such rewards did not come without a price, for *'the* Art of Healing *is never acquir'd but by hard, anxious, and long study, and by accurate Observations.*'[93] Perhaps Charleton was thinking back to the anxiety he endured in 1664 at the hands of

---

88 Ibid., p. 29.

89 Ibid., p. 30.

90 Physiognomy was also part of Charleton's *The Immortality of the Human Soul*. Athanasius assures Lucretius he is pleased to see him to which Lucretius replies: 'Ah! Anthanasius, I am already convinc'd of both. I am not unacquainted with the exteriour Characters of the Passions, as not plainely to perceive the evidences of joy in your countenance. The serenity of your aspect, the pleasant smoothnesse of your forhead, the vivacity and lustre of your eyes, and the unusuall sanguine tincture of your cheeks, are perfect demonstrations of that Passion within you', p. 2.

91 Charleton, *Enquiries*, Preface, p. 13.

92 *Idem.*

93 Ibid., Preface, p. 23.

Scarburgh and Ent, when his anatomical observations proved to be inaccurate and his rational mind had failed him.

These three works of Walter Charleton – one a lively romance, one a meditation on the passions and one a series of lectures to the College of Physicians – have a common theme, the problem of the passions. Charleton believed that the way to curb our most violent sensual responses and acquire the Epicurean virtue of tranquillity of mind, or dispassion, was by gaining anatomical expertise and practising religious virtue. This is perhaps best described as medical Epicureanism. Only then could the seeming dichotomies of body and spirit, emotion and reason, be harmonized.[94] As Charleton exclaimed in the lectures of 1680 '... no Mortal can attain to any profound knowledge of Himself; without long and strict scrutiny into the mysterious Oeconomy of Human nature.'[95] Stories, if told and embellished by anatomists who understood the physiology of the body, could forewarn men of the folly of not controlling their passions. Examining the war within could lead to self-control, even as war and religious strife raged without.

Dissections sculpted not only the bodies of the deceased but also that of the anatomist. They honed the rational mind. Combining knowledge of the body with knowledge of one's self could be used as a philosophical and theological shield against the temptations of a 'passionate breast'. Dispassion entered the emotional community of medical men in various guises. Harvey encountered it in the hospitals of Padua and London, and Samuel Pepys at a banquet in the Barber-Surgeons' Hall. Despite the sight and feel of a wretched corpse, Pepys overcame his emotions and accepted the dispassionate conclusions of a group of doctors, 'that there is no pain at all in hanging, for that it do stop the circulation of the blood, and so stops all sense and motion in an instant.'

94 Winkler, Mary G. (Spring 1993), 'The Anatomical Theater', *Literature and Medicine,* 12 (1), pp. 65–80.

95 Charleton, *Enquiries*, Preface, p. 10.

Chapter Three

Godly Hearts

So that the Knife *and* Lectures *of a skilful* Anatomist*, cannot but preach* Religion *even to the very* Atheist ... [1]

What is called by the Stoics apathy or dispassion; by the Sceptics mean but great tranquility of mind.[2]

An age given over to all vice – whores and harlotts, pimps and panders, bauds and buffoones, lechery and treachery, atheists and papists, rogues and rascalls, reason and treason, playmakers and stageplayers, officers debauched and corrupted (proctor Thomas infected with the pox while proctor) –aggravated and promoted by presbytery.[3]

Conquer thy own passions.[4]

In March 1651 John Evelyn went to see a man being tortured at a prison in Paris:

... they first bound his wrist with a strong rope or small cable, and one end of it to an iron ring made fast to the wall about 4 foote from the floore, and then his feete with another cable, fastened about 5 foote farther than his uttmost length to another ring on the floore of the roome: thus suspended and yet lying but aslant, they slid an horse of wood under the

---

1 Browne, John (1690), *Myographia Nova*, London, p. 31.

2 *The Oxford English Dictionary*, 'Dispassion' from William Temple (1698), *Gardening*. Sir William Temple (1628–99) was a diplomat who negotiated the Triple Alliance of 1688 (Britain, Netherlands and Sweden versus France). He was a friend of John Evelyn with whom he shared a love of gardening. Temple wrote *Upon the Gardens of Epicurus or Of Gardening in the Year 1685*. In 1689 Jonathan Swift became his secretary and Temple would later help him revise 'Tale of a Tub'. Swift made Temple the hero of 'The Battle of the Books'. See Faber, Richard (1983), *The Brave Courtier: Sir William Temple*, London: Faber and Faber, also Marburg, Clara (1932), *Sir William Temple: A Seventeenth Century "Libertin"*, New Haven: Yale University Press, and Shaaber, M.A. (ed). (1957), *Seventeenth Century Prose*, New York: Harper & Brothers Publishers.

3 *The Life and Times of Anthony à Wood* (1961), Oxford: Oxford University Press, p. 130. Wood wrote this on 1 December 1667 shortly after he had taken a vomit 'having bin some dayes before and then possessed with great melancholy and distraction.'

4 Sir D'Arcy Power gave a Presidential Address on 'John Ward and his Diary' in 1916 and again in 1920 to the Medical Society of London. See *Trans. med. Soc. Lond.* (1917), 40, pp. 1–26, reprinted in Sir D'Arcy Power (1931), *Selected Writings*, London, pp. 173–200, and *Trans. med. Soc. Lond*, (1920), 43, pp. 253–84. Power also transcribed the first six volumes of the Diary. See *Transcript of John Ward's Diaries, 1913–26*. Original in The Folger Shakespeare Library with a copy at the Wellcome Library. This quotation is from Power, *Transcript*, p. 65.

> rope which bound his feete, which so exceedingly stiffened it, as seve'd the fellow's joints in miserable sort, drawing him out at length in an extraordinary manner, he having onely a paire of linnen drawers on his naked body: then they questioned him of a robbery.[5]

The prisoner did not confess and the height of the horse was increased. But again there was no confession and the 'Executioner' poured two buckets of water down the man's throat. Evelyn declared that the prisoner's body was then so swollen 'as would have pittied and affrighted any one to see it'. Despite this the man continued to deny the charges and 'What became of him I know not.' Evelyn had fled the prison before the end of the torture even though, 'There was another Malefactor to suceede' and Evelyn was supposed to view his interrogation. But 'the spectacle was so uncomfortable, that I was not able to stay the sight of another.'[6]

The entry in the diary ends with Evelyn trying to make sense of what he had felt while watching the prisoner's pain escalate with each new bout of torture. He had felt sorry for the man and been frightened by the spectacle but above all, 'It represented yet to me, the intolerable sufferings which our Blessed Saviour must need undergo when his body was hanging with all its weight upon the nails on the crosse.'[7] Seeing, hearing and smelling a man endure the rack and water torture had led Evelyn to replace the broken body of the prisoner with the image of the ultimate sufferer for mankind – Jesus Christ. His godly heart had been strengthened by being in the presence of such misery.

Two months later Evelyn went to see the operation for the stone at the Hospital of La Charité in Paris. 'A child of 8 or 9 yeares old underwent the operation with most extraordinary patience, and expressing greate joy when he saw the stone was drawn.' Again, Evelyn focused on the demeanour of the victim and what watching the event meant to him. In this case it was not the sufferings of our Blessed Saviour which came to mind but Evelyn's own fear of the pain of lithotomy. 'The use I made of it was to give Almighty God hearty thankes that I had not ben subject to this deplorable infirmitie.'[8] Again, witnessing another suffer was of 'use' to the onlooker.

Suffering and its relation to religious faith was a constant theme in John Evelyn's *Kalendarium*, as it was in many early modern English diaries and commonplace books. Evelyn recorded the godly behaviour and painful end of his young son in 1658 and his emotional reaction to the death. Evelyn agreed to an autopsy of his son, and felt anger at the cause of death:

> in my opinion he was suffocated by the woman & maide that tended him, & covered him too hott with blankets as he lay in a Cradle, neere an excessive hot fire in a close roome ...

---

5 Bray, William (1819), *Memoirs illustrative of the life and writings of John Evelyn ...* ., London, p. 210.

6 *Idem.*

7 *Idem.* On the *question d'eau*, or water torture, see Silverman, Lisa (2001), *Tortured Subjects: Pain, Truth, and the Body in Early Modern France*, Chicago: University of Chicago Press. She briefly discusses Evelyn on pp. 96–7.

8 Bray, p. 204.

> . Here ends the joy of my life, & for which I go even mourning to the grave: The L. Jesus sanctifie this & all other my Afflictions: Amen:[9]

In March 1670 Evelyn wrote of 'my unspeakeble griefe' at the death of his brother Richard.[10] Poor Richard Evelyn had been in 'such exceeding torture' from the stone and 'all along averse from being cut; but when he at last consented, and it came to the operation and all things prepar'd, his spirit and resolution failed.'[11] During the autopsy a small bladder stone was found. Samuel Pepys, too, was devastated by the end of his brother's life in March 1664:

> I had no mind to see him die, as we thought he presently would, and so withdrew ... [on his return, he was told that his brother had died] I went up and found the nurse holding his eyes shut, and he poor wretch lying with his chops fallen, a most sad sight, and that which put me into a present very great transport of grief and cries.[12]

Obviously, the spectacle of suffering could and did evoke more than pity and empathy. It caused great distress in those who witnessed it. Why then, would some men like John Evelyn seek out opportunities to see operations and witness torture? What was the relationship of pain to religious belief and medical practice? What resources, other than the dispassion that Harvey may have always largely possessed or Charleton's life-long analysis of the passions, could medical men draw on as they operated and dissected? To pose answers to these questions I focus on the life of the clergyman, John Ward (1629–81). Ward jotted down his thoughts, experiences, readings and 'things to do' in 16 notebooks covering 33 years. Often termed his 'Diaries' the volumes are, in fact, largely chronological commonplace books.[13] Sir D'Arcy Power and especially Robert G. Frank have examined Ward's diaries for what they reveal about the community of experimenters at Oxford in the 1650s and early 1660s, and about medicine in general.[14] As is well detailed, Ward participated in dissections and vivisections with Richard Lower, wrote about Thomas Willis's findings on the brain, watched operations and autopsies with local doctors and

---

9 Ibid., pp. 209–10.

10 Ibid., p. 344.

11 *Idem.*

12 Le Galienne, Richard (ed.) (2001), *The Diary of Samuel Pepys*, New York: The Modern Library, p. 122.

13 Miscellaneous extracts were first published by Severn, Charles (1839), *Diary of Rev. John Ward, A.M.*, London.

14 Frank Jr, Robert G., discusses Ward's Diaries from a scientific and medical viewpoint in (1974) 'The John Ward Diaries: Mirror of Seventeenth Century Science and Medicine', *Journal of the History of Medicine*, 49, pp. 147–79. Severn was the only author who included writings in religion or philosophy. Unfortunately as in the case of Power, no citations were included. On Ward see Frank Jr, Robert G. (1994) 'Medicine' in *The History of the University of Oxford*, Vol. IV, Oxford: Oxford University Press. Tyacke, Nicholas (ed.) (1997), *Seventeenth Century Oxford*, pp. 505–58, discusses Ward and the similarity of his commonplace books to John Locke's. Locke collected recipes from Richard Lower and Dr Bathurst of Anne Greene fame, p. 535.

surgeons, visited various chemists and attended public anatomies in London.[15] As a vicar in Stratford-upon-Avon, Ward ministered to the sick in soul and body, collected anecdotes of unusual cases and continued to copy out the latest news on anatomy, mining and chemistry from the *Philosophical Transactions of the Royal Society*.[16]

Besides the appeal of the new philosophy, Ward's commonplace books show the influence of classical authors, especially Seneca, on tempering one's passions. He included excerpts from Thomas Browne's *Religio Medici* and Thomas Fuller's *Andronicus*, 'our English Seneca.' Like William Harvey, John Evelyn and Walter Charleton, John Ward was a staunch Anglican. He copied passages from sermons and religious books into his commonplace book and, in particular, railed against the Quakers who were apparently making headway in Oxford. The focus of this chapter, however, is not on what Ward's writings tell us about the new mechanical philosophy or anatomical discoveries. Rather, it is on what the interplay of the practice of medicine, philosophical interests and religious belief found in Ward's diaries tell us about attitudes towards pain and the passions.

John Ward and the Stoic Body

John Ward was the eldest son of a Northamptonshire rural vicar. His father probably died after being taken prisoner by the Parliamentarians at the Battle of Naseby in 1645.[17] John Ward matriculated at Magdalen College in 1646 and was appointed to a vacant studentship at Church Oxford in 1649 by Parliament's authority.[18] He received his BA in 1649 and MA in 1652, and then stayed in Oxford as a medical student until October 1661. He never took the degree of Bachelor of Medicine. Sometime

---

15 Robert Martensen has written extensively on the relationship of Anatomy to religion in this period. See (1992), '"Habit of Reason": Anatomy and Anglicanism in Restoration England', *Bulletin of the History of Medicine*, 66, pp. 511–35. He gives four reasons for the elite being willing to agree to autopsies: Shared belief in value of learned medicine, at least for their own class, Curiousity itself was gaining positive value among the elite, Important to support the professional and social order, Postmortem manipulation of individuals' earthly remains was not new to privileged families in the Restoration era. I would add a fifth reason – the desire to see the marks of the sufferings in the body and gain comfort from them. On Willis see Martensen (2004), *The Brain Takes Shape: An Early History*, Oxford: Oxford University Press. On Lower and transfusion see Brown, *The Mechanical Philosophy and the 'Animal Oeconomy'*.

16 While Pepys may have been delighted to know the odds of him surviving a lithotomy was recorded in Ward's diaries: 'I was at St. Thomas's Hospital, in Southwerk, the 14th Feb., 1661. The porter told mee that Mr. Holyard cutt 30 of the stone one year, and all lived; and afterwards cutt four, and they all died', Charleton would have smarted at the note in Ward's book that related Scarburgh's anatomical find: 'There was a person dissected att London about October: 1664: who wanted his pectoral Muscles, yet had ye right use of his armes as I heard, wch Dr. Scarborough said was never heard of before.' Severn, p. 235 and John Ward's Diaries, X, 108r.

17 Power, 'John Ward and his Diary', p. 176. The younger son Thomas became rector of Stow-on-the Wold.

18 Frank, 'The John Ward Diaries', p. 148.

in 1660 Ward was ordained, and in 1660 and 1661 the notebooks show that Ward debated whether he should apply for a bishop's licence to practise medicine or obtain an MD from a foreign university. Leiden, Ward noted, charged 16 pounds for an MD, 'besides feasting ye professors'. However, Angiers cost only nine pounds and surprisingly for a French university, 'f[e]asting not necessarie neither'.[19] He spent from 1661 to 1662 visiting the hospitals of Charterhouse, St Bartholomew's and St Thomas' in London and watching operations.[20] But by 1662, Ward had given up the idea of travelling to the Continent, purchased a Lambeth licence for approximately 30 shillings and taken a clerical living at Stratford-upon-Avon. Perhaps the cost of getting an MD was too high? Either way Ward would remain a vicar in Stratford-upon-Avon until his death in 1681. Yet as his writings demonstrate, Ward's interests in the human and animal body, remedies and surgery never waned. He travelled to London and Oxford to buy books, to talk with friends regarding their medical research and to perform his own experiments in anatomy and chemistry.[21]

Was Ward less a reluctant cleric and more a frustrated physician as has been suggested by Power and Frank? It is difficult to tell from his writings. Certainly, throughout his life, Ward continued to jot down thoughts about anatomy and chemistry alongside notes on geography, history and religion. Ward was not unusual in being a cleric with a devotion to medicine.[22] Socially, clergymen and physicians belonged to the same stratum of society, at the lower end of the class of gentlemen but above the men with no true political influence. In terms of career choice, medicine and religion could appear as equal possibilities – as indeed, they did to John Ward.[23] In a sense we have performed a grave disservice in attempting to untangle Ward's scientific and medical entries from the rest of his jottings on religion, philosophy and history. Ward would not, and did not, compartmentalize his life; all was intertwined as it should be. In a popular handbook for clergymen, *A Priest to the Temple, or, The Country Parson* (1652), George Herbert wrote that a cleric should 'desire[s] to be all to his Parish, and not only a Pastour, but a Lawyer also, and a Phisician ... .'[24] Ward's notebooks reflect this appreciation.[25]

---

19 Ward, IX, 117v, 124v–125r.

20 Ward, VIII, 150r–153r and IX, 1r–v.

21 For example, he saw Dr Conyers at Oxford in March 1662, IX, 23v.

22 For a lucid discussion of the relationship of theology to natural philosophy see, Henry, 'The Scientific Revolution in England' in Porter, Roy and Teich, Mikuláš (eds) (1992), *The Scientific Revolution in National Context*, Cambridge and New York: Cambridge University Press. Henry traces the emergence of the Low Church Party or the Latitudinarians from the Great Tew Circle of the 1630s which included Edward Hyde, William Chillingworth, Robert Sanderson, John Hales and Gilbert Sheldon. Their theology of compromise affected natural philosophy, especially after the Restoration.

23 Wear, Andrew (1985), 'Puritan perceptions of illness in Seventeenth-Century England', in Porter, Roy (ed.) *Patients and practitioners: Lay perceptions of medicine in pre-industrial society*, Cambridge and New York: Cambridge University Press, pp. 57–99.

24 Herbert, George (1941), *Works*, ed. Hutchinson, F.E., Oxford: Clarendon Press, p. 259.

25 One of the few places I have found where clerics were cautioned not to practise medicine is: *Popular errours or the errours of the people in matter of Physick: London,1651.*

The appeal of the Church of England to a wide section of the population after the Restoration has been well documented by historians.[26] Fortunately most writers agree on a definition of Anglicanism for the mid seventeenth century:

> The hallmark of Anglicanism ... was the ability to steer a middle course between Rome and Geneva by insisting upon the distinction between what was fundamental for belief and what was not.[27]

> The Restoration Church of England's *via media* between Catholic and Reformed was a broad path, wide enough to accommodate those who wished to hug either side and those who yawed from one to the other.[28]

In a letter of 1671 John Evelyn reflected that for him the appeal of the Anglican Church rested in the sanctuary it provided, 'I found in her alone the *Golden Meane*, neither too streite, nor too wide, but of just dimensions and admirable ... constitution.'[29]

The *via media* or the *Golden Meane* of the Anglican Church was a defensive response to the wars and schisms of the mid seventeenth century and the lures of atheism and materialism after the Restoration. The Church was believed to be surrounded by enemies both at home and abroad. In his customary bilious fashion, Anthony à Wood summed up the prodigious moral and religious ills found just in the city of Oxford alone:

> 1 day, Dec., Su., [1667] I took a vomit, having bin some dayes before and then possessed with great melancholy and distraction.

> An age given over to all vice – whores and harlotts, pimps and panders, bauds and buffoones, lechery and treachery, atheists and papists, rogues and rascalls, reason and treason, playmakers and stageplayers, officers debauched and corrupted (proctor Thomas infected with the pox while proctor) – aggravated and promoted by presbytery.[30]

Translated by Robert Wittie, Doctor in Physick from Latin of James Primrose. Primrose (c.1598–1659) is most famous for opposing Harvey's discovery of the circulation of the blood In 'Chapter IV Of Ministers that Practise Physick', Wittie's translation of Primrose reads, 'for the practise of Physick doth wholly turne away the minde from the study of Divinitie, and the study of Divinitie (in them that preach especially) doth interrupt the practise of Physick; therefore it is very probable, that Physick cannot, with a safe conscience be exercised by any Divine who hath the care of soules.' p. 14.

26 Spurr, John (2003), '"A Sublime and Noble Service": John Evelyn and the Church of England', in *John Evelyn and his Milieu*, Harris, Frances and Hunter, Michael, London: The British Library. The letter is to John Hamilton. On the complex nature of Anglicanism see Spurr (1991), *The Restoration of the Church of England, 1646–1689*, New Haven: Yale University Press, Harris, Tim, Seaward, Paul and Goldie, Mark (eds) (1990), *The Politics of Religion in Restoration England*, London: Blackwell, and Sommerville, C. John (1989) *Popular Religion in Restoration England*, Gainesville FL: University Press of Florida.

27 Henry, p. 192

28 Spurr, *The Restoration Church of England, 1646–1689*, p. 163.

29 Spurr, 'A Sublime', p. 145.

30 *The Life and Times of Anthony à Wood,* p. 130

John Ward, like many ordained ministers in the Church of England, appears to have been a Latitudinarian.[31] The Latitudinarian, or Low Church Party, grew out of the 'Great Tew Circle', which included Edward Hyde, William Chillingworth, Robert Sanderson, John Hales and Gilbert Sheldon. It became the dominant group within the Anglican Church after the Restoration. John Henry succinctly sums up their theology as, 'The aim of Latitudinarianism was to determine the method for establishing the minimum requirements for the true faith.'[32] Martin Griffin has examined the Latitudinarian theory of knowledge and describes it as resting in the belief that there 'was an essential harmony between the mind and reality.'[33] This harmony found its expression in 'the light of nature', a phrase which recurs time and again in the writings of the Great Tew Circle:

> Belief in the light of nature presumed a static, orderly external reality governed by law, whether moral or 'natural'; because it was governed by law, it was therefore accessible to human reason.'[34]

The notion of the 'light of nature' had long roots which stretched back to ancient philosophy, particularly Stoicism.

Like Epicureanism, Stoicism was revived during the Renaissance by humanists interested in classical languages.[35] The affinity of Stoicism to Christianity was noted both in terms of its ideology and in the belief that life during the turbulent Counter-Reformation was much like what the Stoics had experienced in the crumbling Roman Empire.[36] One of the most important agents in the transmission of Roman Stoicism to England was the Leiden professor of history and law, Justus Lipsius (1547–1606).[37] Lipsius, a Belgian classical philologist and Humanist, wrote several works with the aim of reviving Stoicism in a form that would be compatible with Christianity. The triad of *constantia, patientia, firmitas*, (constancy, patience, firmness) was first developed by Lipsius in his *De Constantia Libri Duo, Qui alloquium praecipue continent in Publicis malis* (1584). It was translated into English four times between

---

31 Severn, *passim.*

32 Henry, p. 193.

33 Griffin, JR., Martin I.J. (1992), *Latitudinarianism in the Seventeenth Century Church of England*, Leiden: Brill Academic Publishers, p. 68.

34 *Idem.*

35 Seneca was often lumped in with Epicurus and vice versa. See Fothergill-Payne, Louise (1991), 'Seneca's role in popularizing Epicurus in the sixteenth century', in Osler, Margaret, (ed.), *Atoms, pneuma, and tranquillity*, Cambridge and New York: Cambridge University Press, pp. 115–33. In the same volume see Barker, Peter, 'Stoic contributions to early modern science', pp. 135–54. Also Proctor, Judith (1995), *The Suffering Self: Pain and Narrative Representation in the Early Christian Era*, New York and London: Routledge.

36 Oestreich, Gerhard, Oestreich, Brigitta and Koenigsberger, H.G. (eds) (1982), *Neostoicism and the early modern state*, trans. McLintock, David, Cambridge and New York: Cambridge University Press, p. vii.

37 On Justus Lipsius see Evans, Robert C. (1992), *Jonson, Lipsius and The Politics of Renaissance Stoicism*, Wakefield, N.H.: Longwood Academic, and Morford, Mark (1991), *Stoics and Neostoics: Rubens and the Circle of Lipsius*, Princeton: Princeton University Press.

1594 and 1670. In 1605 Lipsius brought out a new critical edition of Seneca's *Omnia opera* and became the first to popularize Roman Stoicism in general and Seneca in particular.[38]

Lipsius sharply criticised *miseratio,* or pity, as being of no use to man and called for, 'an exceedingly severe, controlled manliness in the Stoic mold, in short for a character anchored in reason.'[39] Emotions were the product of mere opinions (opinio) and led to distress and imbalance. A man must analyze and reject his opinions using reason (*ratio*). This will free him from the inconstancy that the passions bring. Thomas Lodge published the first English edition of Seneca's essays in 1614 as *The Workes of Lucius Annaeus Seneca Newly Inlarged and Corrected by Thomas Lodge, D.M.P.* In a chapter titled 'Of his sicknesses', Lodge explained that for the Stoics, 'our paine is but an opinion' and drew a correlation between sickness and torture:

> Tell me how whatsoever thou wilt, both of the discent of Rhumes, and of the vertue of a continuall cough, that maketh a man yeeld up a part of his bowels, and of a fevor that scorcheth the intrailes, and of thirst and of the joynts of feete and hands, which griefe and paine hath contracted and dislocated. The flame, the racke, the burning and glowing plates, and that which is laid upon the swollen wounds, to renue their paine, and to make it pierce more deepe, is yet more cruell.[40]

All of this misery could be endured by a true Stoic:

> And yet there has beene some, that have suffered all this without complaining. It is a small matter. And hath not once besought them to give over. It is a toy. And that hath never answered. It is a trifle. That hath laughed out-right with all his heart. After all this, wilt thou laugh at paine?[41]

Pain and torture were like the passions. They were perturbations or perilous forces that acted on the suffering body.[42] To be a Stoic, or in the case of the seventeenth century, a NeoStoic, required a man to exercise self-control when experiencing pain inwardly, having it applied to him outwardly, or witnessing others in pain. All pain is equal in what is expected of the Stoic, he is to be dispassionate or pitiless.

By 1640 'Stoicall apathists who are insensible of passion' were being mocked in poems,[43] and there is strong evidence that NeoStoicism held an appeal for

38 Oestreich, p. 14.

39 Ibid., p. 29.

40 Lodge, Thomas (1614), *The Workes of Lucius Annaeus Seneca Newly Inlarged and Corrected by Thomas Lodge, D.M.P, London,* Vol. II, p. 319. On the difficulty of describing the experience of pain see Scarry, Elaine (1985), *The Body in Pain*, Berkeley: University of California Press, 1985, and Rey, Roselyne (1993), *History of Pain*, trans. Wallace, Louise Elliott, Cadden J.A. and Cadden, S.W., Paris: Editions la Decouverte.

41 Lodge, Vol. II, p. 319.

42 Paster, Gail Kern, Rowe, Katherine, Floyd-Wilson, Mary (eds) (2004), *Reading the Early Modern Passions,* Introduction.

43 *Oxford English Dictionary*, 'Apathist: One addicted to apathy, one sunk in stolid indifference, Apathy was the highest state of humanity according to the Stoics. Richard

educated men.[44] Such commonplace books of seventeenth-century Oxford and Cambridge students, for example, are littered with passages from Seneca.[45] Educated Latitudinarians were prominent contributors to discussions of Stoic thought. John Wilkins, for example, in his *Principles and Duties of Natural Religion*, by lengthy and frequent quotations from the Stoic sages Seneca, Lucan, Musonius, Epictetus and Marcus Aurelius, permitted them to say almost as much as he did himself.[46]

John Ward's notebooks are peppered with quotations from Seneca, lists of books on the passions he should buy, and Stoic-like reminders on the danger of violent feelings. In 1648 we find:

> 'Remembr YT I peruse Senecas works with diligence and plutarchs livs and morals', 'It is the method of charity to suffer without reaction', 'We naturally know what is good but naturally prefer what is evill. Sense must sit at the feet of Reason'[47] and 'Conquer thy own passions.'[48]

Sixteen years later, he again mentioned Seneca as well as a list of favoured authors:

> 'Remember to get Tullie and Seneca handsome pleasant Books frequently to peruse.' 'Remember to buy Lucretius if I have him not and to peruse Mr Farringdons Sermons and B. Brownrigg's: and to buy Senault on ye passions and some character men.'[49]

In 1666 Ward once again reminded himself that 'Violent passions are like an unruly horse that runs away with a man, and stopps neither at river nor precipice.'[50]

What made Stoicism of interest to John Ward, especially as he began to dissect and vivisect, may have been its stress on reason and self-control. Within the belief system of NeoStoics, pain was a bodily manifestation irrelevant to the noble and spiritual life. It must be controlled by the mind and endured by the body. Viewed through this lens, Aurelius Celsus's oft-repeated advice on the surgeon's demeanour towards the suffering patient becomes perfectly sensible. James Cooke, a Warwick

---

Brathwait, Boulster lecture 216, 1640. Brathwait (*d*.1673) was a poet and playwright. His best known work is (1631), *The English Gentlewoman*.

44 For an excellent analysis of Christianized Stoic ethics, see Cunningham, Andrew (1996), 'Sir Thomas Browne and Religio Medici', in Grell, Ole Peter and Cunningham, Andrew (eds), *Religio Medici: Medicine and Religion in Seventeenth-Century England*, London: Scolar Press, pp. 12–61.

45 Todd, Margo (1983), 'Seneca and the Protestant Mind: The Influence of Stoicism on Puritan Ethics', in *Archiv fur Reformationsgeschichte*, 74, pp. 182–99. Even Thomas Wharton, a confirmed Aristotelian included a quotation from Seneca on the title page of *Adenographia*. 'Veniet tempus, quo ista quæ nunc latent, in lucem dies extrabat & longioris ævi diligentia.' Freer translates this as, 'There will come a time when things that are now obscure will be brought to light by the dawn of a new day, and as a result of diligent research over a longer period of time.' Freer, Stephen and Cunningham, Andrew (eds) (1996), *Thomas Wharton's Adenographia*, Oxford: Clarendon Press.

46 Griffin, p.70.

47 Ward, I 18v.

48 Power, *Transcript*, p. 65.

49 Ibid., pp. 613, 616, 675.

50 Ward, IV 146v.

surgeon, urged young surgeons in *Mellificium Chirurgiae* (1685) to follow the advice of Celsus and be '*Pitiless*, as not by clamor, either to overhasten or forbear his work more than necessity requires in the Cure under hand.'[51] The enthusiasm for NeoStoicism may explain to some extent why this phrase crops up again and again in later sixteenth- and seventeenth-century surgical works.[52] In Stoicism, pity was a useless emotion, it simply made the onlooker feel as wretched and pathetic as the sufferer. This was considered irrational and so the Stoic sought to control his emotions and not be disturbed by others' pain:

> Seneca maintained the sapiens 'would perform precisely the same actions as someone feeling pity, and would simply do so while controlling his feelings, with a tranquil mind, without causing himself misery: he will bring relief to another's tears, he will not add his own'.[53]

The elevation of right reason in NeoStoicism and the peace it brought to the mind was attractive to Anglicans who walked the *via media.* Both the philosophy and the religion emphasized control over the self, fortitude, resilience and the acceptance of one's fate. Anglicans identified their religious foes (Quakers, Calvinists and Catholics) as lacking this tranquil mind.[54]

Atheists were another kettle of fish. They were the antithesis of the rational constant NeoStoic. Walter Charleton explicitly equated atheism with the loss of reason and portrayed atheists as subhuman – 'beasts':

> *... we may safely conclude, that to study Anatomy diligently and reverently, is to learn to know God, and consequently to venerate Him;* Deum enim colit, qui novit ... *this I openly declare, that if I knew an* Atheist *(if there be such a Beast in the world) I would do my best to bring him into this Theatre, here to be sensibly convinced of his madness.*[55]

While anatomists such as Molinetti and Vesling at Padua had claimed that cutting and viewing the body brought one closer to God as the body was a microcosm of the macrocosm, the claim that witnessing a dissection might even convert an atheist was new because the concept of atheism was new. Even Charleton seemed to have a hard time imagining such 'a beast' and he had come perilously close to being branded one. (One wonders if there were any sniggers in the Anatomy Theatre as Charleton appeared to struggle with the *very idea* of an atheist.)

This theme of anatomy being a cure for this imaginary group of atheists appeared to come to fruition after the Restoration with the concern for political and social

51 Cooke, James (1685), *Mellificium Chirurgiae: Or, The Marrow of Chirurgery. An Anatomical Treatise*, London, p. 1. This was the fourth edition.

52 See Wear, Andrew (2000), *Knowledge and practice in English Medicine,1550–1680*, Cambridge and New York: Cambridge University Press, pp. 216, 222, 240–42.

53 Proctor, p. 88.

54 In 1688 John Evelyn was willing to extend 'Indulgence to all sober dissenters; Socinians, Independents, & Quakers (in my owne Judgment) to be excepted: I am sure the first are scarsly Christian, & the latter of publique danger & unaccountable'. Spurr, 'A Sublime', p. 156.

55 Charleton, *Enquiries*, the Preface, p. 16. Italics in original.

order; it lasted throughout the seventeenth century. John Browne, a surgeon at St Thomas' included this address from Edmund Dickinson, a physician to Charles II and James II, in *Myographia Nova: Or, A Graphical Description of All the Muscles in the Human Body as they arise in Dissection* (1690):

> *So that the* Knife *and* Lectures *of a skilful* Anatomist, *cannot but preach* Religion *even to the very* Atheist, *when he sees the stupendious* Make of Living Creatures, *when he considers the* Subtilty, *the* Variety, *and wise Contrivance of* Parts *in the most minute, as well as in the largest Animals, by which all their inward and outward Actions and Motions, their Sounds, their Voices and Words were formed and exerted. All which, nothing less than an* Omnipotent Being *could effect.*[56]

Words and knives were the weapons of anatomists when it came to revealing the wonders of the body and God's design for mankind. Martin Griffin compared the style and language of the sermons of the Latitudinarians to the style and language of the Royal Society. The Latitudinarians were meant to speak in 'familiar terms' and avoid 'all literary artifices, particularly metaphors' and organize 'their sermons methodically, dividing them into clearly defined subtopics, and concluding them with a summary and application.'[57] Similarly, quoting from Thomas Sprat:

> ... the Fellows of the Royal Society studied: 'to reject all amplifications, digressions, and swellings of style: to return back to the primitive purity, and shortness, when men delivered so many *things*, almost in an equal number of *words*. They have exacted from their members, a close, naked, natural way of speaking; positive expressions; clear senses; a native easiness; bringing all things as near the mathematical plainness as they can.[58]

Michael Hunter argues that the early members of the Royal Society did attempt to set themselves apart from the 'enthusiasm of the sectarians and Puritans and the materialism of the atheists'.[59] John Henry concurs with Griffin that style and words were to be the weapons in this war. The new image and the new way of doing science after the Restoration were spurred on by reforms in the Church of England that focused on language. Dogma, disputations and arguments had led to wars:

> Providing we accept, however, that the link between religion and natural philosophy did not depend upon a particular set of theological doctrines but rather on a method of arriving

---

56 Browne, *Myographia Nova,* p. 31. In 1667 Anthony à Wood attacked Dr Dickinson for his treatment of Mary Woode's pain in her right hip, 'This is to be noted that the doctor did extreamly erre in managing the cure, and did, as "twere, kill her downe-right."' Wood gloated, 'And this was the doctor she loved and doted on soe much as so great, learned, and well-deserving, phisitian!' *The Life and Times of Anthony à Wood,* pp. 165–6.

57 Griffin, p. 136.

58 *Idem*, quotation from Sprat, Thomas (1667), *History of the Royal Society*, London, p. 113.

59 See Hunter, Michael (1981), *Science and Society in Restoration England*, Cambridge and New York: Cambridge University Press, and Shapin, S. and Schaffer, S. (1989), *Leviathan and the Air-Pump*, Princeton: Princeton University Press, on the challenges of atheism to natural philosophers. Also Hooke, Robert (1665), *Micrographia*, London, especially the Preface, and Sprat, *History of the Royal Society.*

at the 'safe way to salvation' we can see the more general affiliation between science and religion.[60]

It is now time to consider what language John Ward used in writing about the body, the passions and his godly heart.

John Ward and the kitchen body

In early 1660 Ward recorded first the illness and then his attendance at the autopsy of one of his fellow college members, Edmund Gwynne:

> Mr Gwinne of our house vomited up long pieces of blood wch had heads like fishes. They carried them to the Apothecaries and cut them but knew not what to make of them ... I saw Mr Gwinne of our house dissected, but could perceive nothing in him that might cause his death; his spleen was somewhat flaccid, so was his heart, and one of his kidnies ... they pretended hee had a contusion of the liver, in regard ye concavity of itt was a little stained or possibly itt was nothing else but the settling of ye blood when death came. There was a membrane coming from his side to his lungs on each side wch some ignorant people would have interpreted a growing of ye lungs to ye side, but Mr. Boghill said he had seen it severall times in sound men YT hee had opened. His heart was large, about as large as ye heart of an ox but not perisht at all.[61]

In the autopsy of Mr Gwynne, animal anatomy appears to have been a reference point for human structure. The animal imagery is notable (the fish heads and ox heart) and may reflect Harvey's popularization of comparative anatomy among Ward's acquaintances: Thomas Willis, Richard Lower, Robert Boyle and Walter Needham. Harvey certainly used such imagery in describing the poor laundress's prolapsed uterus as being like a 'Bull's Cod'.[62]

Not surprisingly, as a keen student of medicine, Ward quickly separated his knowledge of anatomy from that of 'ignorant people' and noted what Mr Boghill, a local apothecary, had to say. While the autopsy seems to have been less than successful in determining a cause of death, Ward's description says a great deal about the procedure and his approach to the body. In this case and many others, he frequently uses animal or plant terminology to describe substances that come out of body orifices or that are seen post-mortem. During and after surgery, and in dissection, Ward describes flesh and fluid being skilfully sliced, boiled, distilled and preserved. Fluids are measured in buckets, flagons and porringers.

Two other cases, those of a woman who died from dropsy and another from a breast tumour, further illustrate Ward's combination of the educated and the commonplace in his writings. Some remarks are technically descriptive and others

60 Henry, p. 199.

61 Ward, VII. 30r. Power states that this was Edmund Gwynne, a servitor, who matriculated at Christ Church in 1655 and was under the care of Dr Dickenson, Linacre Lecturer at Oxford and of Eton and Merton Colleges. Robert Boyle was also present at the autopsy. 'John Ward and his Diary', p. 194.

62 See Chapter One.

seem comfortably domestic. In May 1661 Ward acted as assistant to Dr William Conyers, a physician in Oxford, as he supervised the opening of a woman who had died of dropsy:

> [We] found very strange things. Her liver and stomach and her duodenum, and some other of her intestines, with her kidneys were got up into her breast, and that without any dilaceration of the diaphragm.[63]

This was a far more satisfying experience because unlike in the case of Mr Gwynne, Ward saw anatomical abnormalities that suggested a cause of death. He watched and may well have helped Conyers collect, boil and inspect the fluid hauled out of the corpse in buckets:

> Dr Conyers took out of the woman's bellie three buckets full of water, and afterwards went about to distill a good deal of itt, but hee found very little of itt rise, not above three or four spoonfulls, the rest when itt settled turnd to a kind of slime or mucilage when itt was cold.[64]

Autopsies were popular events, particularly, when they revealed such interesting anatomy, 'Dr Lydall saied hee would have given forty shillings to have seen itt ....'[65]

In 1667 Ward witnessed the standard early modern method of removing a breast cancer from Mrs Townshend. A small incision was made and fingers used to detach the mammary gland bluntly from the thoracic wall, until in the end only a rim of skin had to be cut.[66] Ward carefully observed the manual technique of the surgeons, their joint manipulation of the physical body, their handling of instruments and the scant loss of blood:

> A cancer in Mrs Townsend's Breast of Alverston taken off by two surgeons .... First they cutt ye skinne cross and laid itt back, yn they workt their hands in ytt one above and the other below and so till their hands mett and so brought itt out. They had their needles and waxt thread ready but never ust them and allso their cauterising irons, but they used them not. Shee lost not above six ounces in all.[67]

---

63 Ward, VIII, 65r. Mr Gill an Oxford surgeon was the one who cut the body open while Drs Conyers and Levins watched. Surgeons appear to have regularly conducted post-mortems. Ward records post mortems by Francis Smith, William Day, John Gill and Roger Fry. Fry was the 'Anatomist of the University' according to James Yonge. He showed Yonge the rarities where the public dissections were held, *The Journal of James Yonge*, p. 181. When Day died in 1665, Fry conducted the autopsy and Ward recorded that Fry told him Day 'had a hole in one kidney so large YT one might turne ones finger in itt; he died of a dropsie'. See Ward, VII 52r, XI 17v and XI 63r.

64 *Idem.*

65 *Idem.*

66 See De Moulin, Daniel (1983), *A Short History of Breast Cancer*, Boston: Martinus Nijhoff Publishers Group, pp. 17–31.

67 Ward, II 98r.

Ward then moved from the patient being operated on to operating on the tumour. Dr Walter Needham had rushed to see the operation but missed it. Instead he arrived in time to diagnose the tumour as being a 'Meliceris' or a large fluid filled sac. It was then cut into pieces and carefully preserved in wine and spices much as fruit would be:

> Dr Needham coming too late staied ye next day to see it opened. Hee said itt was a Meliceris, and not a perfect cancer, but it would have been one quickly. There came out a flow of a great quantitie of waterish substance, as much as would fill a flaggon; when they had done, they cutt off one one bitt, another another, and putt in a glass of wine and some lint, and so lett itt alone untill the next day; then they opend itt again and injected myrrhe, aloes, and such thing as resisted putrefecation, and so bound itt upp againe.[68]

Ward appears to have attended several of Mrs Townshend's dressing changes and further amputations of the cancerous growth. Like John Evelyn, he carefully observed the demeanour of the patient:

> Every time they drest itt, they cutt off something of the cancer that was left behind; the chyrurgions were for applying a caustick, but Dr. Needham said no, not till the last, since shee could endure the knife. They prepard her bodie somewhat, and let her blood the day before. Shee endured itt with infinite patience all along not offering to lay her hand uppon itt to ease itt but a warme cloth to ye other breast all ye time. One of the chyrurgeons told her afterwards, that shee had indured soe much, YT hee would have lost his life ere hee would have sufferd ye like; and ye Dr said hee had read YT women would indure more yn men, but did not beleeve itt till yn.[69]

As in the case of John Evelyn, Ward marvelled at the bravery of some patients as they 'endured the knife' and probably agreed with the surgeon that he could not have put up with the pain Mrs Townshend did. A few months after the operation she died and Ward returned to dissect her with a local surgeon. There is a breathless quality about this passage and this, along with the fact that he and Mr Eedes did not bring 'things convenient' such as sponges to soak up fluid when the body was opened, suggest they may have raced to get to the body first:

> 1668 Mrs. Townsend, of Alverston, being dead of a cancer, Mr. Eedes and I opened her breast in the outward part, and found itt very cancrous; itt had been broken, and a mellicerous part was yet remaining when wee saw itt, which being launct, yielded two porringers full of a very yellow substance, which came out plentifully out of the cavities of the breast. The flesh that was growne againe, after part was taken out, was of a hard gristly substance, which seemed very strange. The ribbs were not putrefied as wee could discerne, not anything within the breast of a cancrous nature, for wee runne the knife withinside the breast through the intercostal muscles. Dr Needham has affirmed that a cancer is much within as without the breast, and hee hath seen a string, as I was told, going from the breast to the uterus. I suppose itt was the mamillarie veins full of knotts which were cancrous, and hung much like ropes of onions. The cancer was a strange one,

68 Ibid. 98v.

69 Ibid. 99v.

as was evident; wee wanted spunges and other things convenient, or else wee had opened the cavitie of the breast.[70]

In all three cases – Mr Gwynne, the woman with dropsy and Mrs Townshend – John Ward employed a curious mixture of mundane and learned terms in his entries. Mr Gwynne vomited up blood like 'fish heads' and had a 'flaccid spleen' and a 'membrane', the woman had 'buckets of water' removed and a 'duodenum', Ward imagined cancerous 'mamillarie veins' as 'ropes of onions'. At autopsy Mrs Townshend's body yielded up 'porringers' of fluid. No doubt, the dissections Ward attended and assisted at were done on kitchen tables with flagons and porringers at hand. Many other examples could be given, but hopefully these three demonstrate the style in which Ward wrote about sickness and dissections.[71] When it came to observing the body in sickness and in death Ward placed his experiences and emotions within the two worlds which he was most comfortable with; first, the professional one of medicine with its anatomical nomenclature and learned explanations of disease; second, the domestic one with its manual labour and household ingredients. One enabled him to view the body as a place of learned knowledge, the other to see the body as a locus of mundane and measurable activity. Ward was not alone in this approach.

Certainly, surgical texts of the seventeenth century can read in parts like elaborate cookbooks. In *Mellificium Chirurgiae* (1685) James Cooke, a surgeon and physician in Warwick gave instructions on how to prepare a skeleton. His title aptly translates as the 'Marrow of Surgery'. First Cooke wrote, 'boil the bones for four or five hours, then scrape and clean them while they are hot. After scraping, the bones should be boiled again for an hour and then left to whiten in the air for two to three months.'[72] William Cowper, an Oxford surgeon, gave instructions in *The Anatomy of Humane Bodies* (1698) on how to skin and boil a heart so the fibres can be seen. First, take off any major blood vessels, next, evacuate the blood:

... then with Tow, or Pieces of Rags, fill the Ventricles, Auricles, and large Vessels on the Basis of the Heart: the Mouths of the large Blood-Vends being stitch'd up, least their Contents should be Extruded by the Contraction of the Heart in Boyling.[73]

Cooking times were provided for animal and human preparations, 'if it is the Heart of an Ox etc. Boyl it Four or Five Hours: if of a Man, One or Two.'[74] This is skilled work and Cowper helpfully provided his readers with a copper plate showing how the human heart should look after you had finished stuffing, stitching and boiling it

70 Ibid., XII 32v. Frank, 'Medicine' in *The History of the University of Oxford*, states that autopsies became more frequent mid century. 'Lower, Millington and Willis did a particularly spectacular post-mortem in May 1666 on the body of a young Wadham scholar struck by lightning while aboard a rowing boat on the Thames. John Wallis reported that despite the hot weather and close room, at least 40 attended.' p. 548.

71 See Ward, IV, 13r, 30r and X *passim.*

72 Cooke, p. 347.

73 Cowper, William (1698), *The Anatomy of the Human Body*, London, Figure 2.

74 *Idem.*

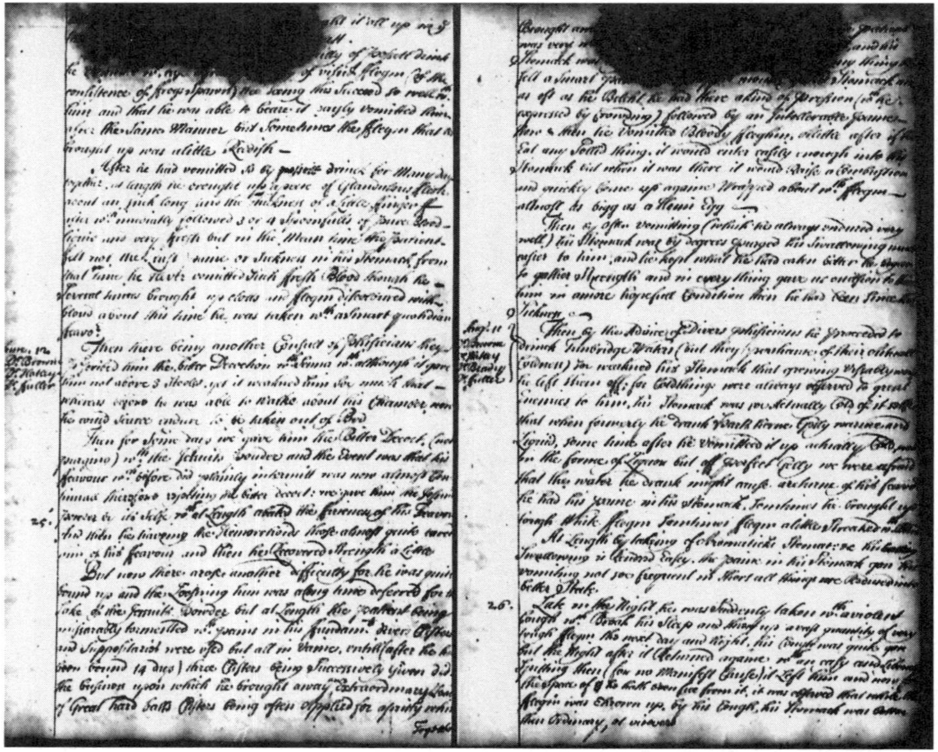

Figure 3.1 Grace (Randolph) Blome, *Her Booke*, 1697, 2nd page of the account of her father's illness/autopsy, V.b.301. By permission of the Folger Shakespeare Library.

up. It is also unpleasant and disturbing work requiring great concentration and an ability to deal with the body on a primitive level as a piece of meat, at least for a while.[75]

As Ward witnessed in Oxford and Evelyn in Paris, surgery was painful to watch as well as to bear. It also caused pain in the operator. James Cooke described removing a dead child in pieces from the womb as 'dreadful'. His account of using a hook to pry out a foetus is indeed dreadful to read:

> At *Kennelworth* four miles from *Warwick*, I fixed my Instrument on the Childs Neck, both the Arms having been pull'd off before I came. After it had at twice or thrice divided the Flesh, at last it fell on the Bones, and in drawing, the Neck broke quite off, and finding the Shoulders come, I fixed again, and brought the Body away; and presently putting up my Hand, and getting hold on the Mouth, I brought the Head away ... .[76]

A striking example of the connection of the world of the kitchen to the world of medicine is found in a manuscript belonging to Grace Blome (1674–1750) from Sevenoaks, Kent. Grace's book, written in 1697, is a cookbook. It contains nearly 500 recipes for everything from mince pies to venison and suet puddings that Grace had collected over time. The final pages of the cookbook are devoted, however, to a long and careful description of her father's illness, death and autopsy in 1684.[77]

Much of it is copied from the doctors's reports of his illness and findings on death. It reads as a chronology of what John Blome ate, drank, coughed up, vomited and excreted and, finally, what substances were found in his body post-mortem as a result of all this tormented activity. The descriptions are similar to Ward's in their vivid comparisons of human anatomy and physiology with animals and household items.

Grace's father, John Blome, was 'very Fatt and lusty (but accounted some what Spleanatick) being also usually troubled wth a flux of Blood ...' from hæmorrhoids.[78] In the hard winter of 1683 he developed a dry cough and fever and eventually travelled to London in April 1684 where he underwent a course of 'Phisick'. This sent him into a decline and he vomited 'a great quantity ... (of the consistence of frogs Spawn)' and 'glandulous flesh'.[79] His phlegm was 'almost as bigg as a Henn Egg'.[80] On the advice of Drs Fuller and Needham he was put on a 'Milk Dyet'. He then 'vomitted 2 Littel pieces of flesh hardly soe bigg as a grain of Wheat wch. at first were Bloody and very Red, but being put into a vial full of Faire Water they quickly

75 Wear, *Knowledge & Practice in English Medicine*, discusses early modern surgical instructions on how to amputate as resembling 'how to joint a piece of meat', p. 252.

76 Cooke, p. 170. Wilson, Adrian (1995), *The Making of Man-midwifery: Childbirth in England, 1660–1770*, Cambridge, MA: Harvard University Press, pp. 49–53 briefly discusses Cooke's obstetrical cases.

77 Grace (Randolph) Blome, *Her Booke*, 1697, V.b. 301, The Folger Shakespeare Library. Grace had 12 children and died at the ripe old age of 76. The account of her father's illness and death is five pages long and unpaginated. I have numbered them ff.1–5 for ease of citation.

78 Blome, f. 1.

79 Ibid., f .2.

80 Ibid., f. 3.

grew white and seem'd to be of a Glandulous contexture ... .'[81] By September John Blome was vomiting 'white digested Matter (like Snott) ...' and a black liquid.[82] Two days after his death his body was opened by 'Dr. Fuller Mr. Nicols assisting':

1. Although he accounted Spleanatick yet his Splean was very sound both as to the Colour and Substancc of it –
2. His Liver was of the same Redness it ought to be and Seemed – altogether Sound –
3. But his Gall Blader was full of Stones (when they put them in liquid, gave a yellow tincture to the water)
4. His Lungs were without fault …
5. Out of a Certaine Veine, a Little above the Lungs grew a Piece of polipous flesh .9 Inches Long
6. The lower part of the Oesophagus and the Upper part of the Stomack were full of fleshy growths which ... by Stopping the passage caused the difficulty of Swallowing ... the worst of flesh were soe pulvisied and Tender that they might be Squeezed to pieces between ones fingers & Thumbs & the parts whereto they grew were something Black and Soe much Corrupted YT one might pass ones finger through them –
7. His Stomack was too plaine, and destitute of folds and mucilaginious fleghm –
   But this was Miraculous that though through the whole Sickness of the patient, he vomitted rough Phlegm and Blood, and also in the very night he died Black matter, we could find no Reliques or Signes of those only probing a vein that was a little Blacker than ordinary wth. my finger, forcing it forwards it oozed a little blood into the Stomack –.[83]

As in the case of Mr Gwynne, the woman with dropsy and Mrs Townshend, John Blome's body was probed with fingers and pieces were removed to be examined and tested. What the two medical men searched for, however, was not the cause of death but rather, to discern how the suffering John Blome endured was manifested in his body after death. In other words they were seeking an explanation of his pain not in the patient but for the family and themselves. They found his stomach was blocked off by fleshy growths so that is why he could hardly swallow. But despite the patient's constant vomiting, Dr Fuller and Mr Nicols found little of the vomit in the body. This was deemed miraculous, as poor John Blome appeared to have been a fountain of vomit from the account of the doctors.

Similarly, John Evelyn appeared to take comfort from the autopsy of his son as a means to explain his son's sufferings rather than the cause of death. As previously noted, Evelyn believed his son had been suffocated by the servants. The diarist 'suffered' to have the boy opened so he could obtain an explanation of the pain they had all endured, his son physically and his family emotionally:

> I sufferd the Physitians to have him opened: Dr. *Needham* & Dr. *Welles* ... Being open'd they found a membranous substance growing to the cavous part of the *liver*, somewhat neere the edge of it for the compasse of 3 Inches, which ought not to be; for the Liver is fixed onely by three strong ligaments, all far distant from that part, insomuch as it could not move in that part; on which they confidently affirm'd, the Child was (as tis vulgarly

81 Ibid., f. 3.
82 Ibid., f. 4.
83 Ibid., f. 5.

> cald) *liver-growne*, & thence that sicknesse & so frequent complaint of his side: & indeede both *Liver* & *Splen* were exceedingly large &c:[84]

John Evelyn's painstaking description of his son's autopsy in his diary; Grace Blome's careful preservation of the history of the illness, death and autopsy of her father in her cookbook; and John Ward's accounts of disease and dissection intermingled with notes on history and religion in his commonplace books share common elements. As in surgeons' instructions on how to prepare specimens and pull out a dead foetus, the emphasis is on manual dexterity, careful measurement and a vision of the body as a repository of wonders and horrors, some explicable and others not:

> Goodie Mylword beyond ye Bridg brought mee ye bagge of an Imposthume wch came from her Daughter or Neece, ye thickest YT ever I saw: ye wench hath felt itt long under her left Breast and itt bled and trickled very warme as shee thought but about 9 days agoe ceased. This morning shee was taken with a Reatching and att last up comes a quart of blood and after ye Bagge wch Mrs. Tyler caught hold of and brought up and was very thick. The question is whether itt comes from her Breast or not or whence itt should come. Itt is probably a vein was opened in her breast by straining herself to take up a payl and se ye water collected and Imposthumated.[85]

John Ward's 16 volumes of notes give us glimpses of how a Restoration Anglican vicar with an interest in classical philosophy, a passion for medicine and a love of history responded to the sufferings of others. Adrian Johns writes that:

> ... physicians dealt with the body, ministers –'spiritual physicians' – with the soul. Both, though, could and did feel themselves qualified to discourse of a branch of knowledge which, traversing the gulf separating the body from soul, embraced *embodied* morality … This was what they meant when they discoursed of the 'passions'.[86]

Religion and medicine were linked by the passions. It is where the two overlapped and sometimes collided. In Paris John Evelyn focused on his bodily response to the torture of the body of a prisoner and made use of the passions it elicited to come closer to the body of Christ on the cross. James Cooke provided a picture of obstetric surgery, summing it up as dreadful but necessary. Grace Blome and her family wanted to witness her father's suffering post-mortem by having his corpse opened, and they saw a miracle in his body. John Ward described disease and dissections in the languages of medicine and domesticity. His matter-of-fact accounts of human suffering evidence a dispassion, shaped by the revival of NeoStoicism after a period of religious wars and the power of Latitudinarianism.

---

84 De Beer, E.S. (1959), *The Diary of John Evelyn, Kalendarium*, Oxford: Clarendon Press, Vol. III, pp. 209–10. Evelyn's son was just 3 years old. He erected a monument to him in St Nicholas's Church, Deptford. The entry is 30 January 1658. In February, 'The afflicting hand of God being still upon us, it pleased him also to take away from us this morning my other youngest sonn *George* now 7 weekes languishing at Nurse, breeding Teeth, & ending in a Dropsie: Gods holy will be don ... .' 3, p. 210.

85 Powers, *Transcript*, 3, p. 571.

86 Johns, Adrian (1996), 'The Physiology of Reading and the Anatomy of Enthusiasm', in *Religio Medici*, pp. 136–70. Quotation from p. 146.

Given the close intellectual, social and practical links between religion and medicine, it is not surprising that they were sometimes viewed as one and the same in terms of the virtues required of even their less learned practitioners – surgeons. In 1686 an anonymous translator of Jan Muys's *A rational practice of chyrurgery* addressed the reader:

> In Physick and Chyrurgery the Case is the same, as in Divinity. For there are some whose Faith is so streight-laced that if you ask them the Grounds therof, ther Answer will be; They believe as the Church believes; and so there's an end of the Argument. But others there are who are not contented with this Implicite Faith, their Religion being grounded on right Reason and Experience. Such is the true Chyrurgeon, that maketh not the least Application to any part or Member of the Body, but can give a Reason Anatomically (or distinctly) why and wherefore he doth the same: otherwise he deserves not so much as the Name of Surgeon.[87]

What was 'Right Reason' in faith and medicine was a question that occupied many in the seventeenth century. Equally, the question of how to maintain control in the face of 'Experience' led to many answers. Reflecting on all the philosophies he had heard of in his lifetime that sought to help one subdue the passions, the diplomat and Epicurean William Temple wrote:

> What is called by the Stoicks Apathy, or Dispassion; by the Scepticks, Indisturbance; by the Molinists, Quietism; by common men, Peace of Conscience; seems all to mean but great Tranquility of Mind, though it be made to proceed from so diverse Causes, as Human, Wisdom, Innocence of Life, or Resignation to the Will of God.[88]

The list is long and reflects the turbulence of Temple's century and the desire on men's part to find a means of controlling their responses to pain in their lives. A godly heart was one that accepted the miseries of life and that acquired peace through the exercise of reason and conscience. Sadly when the surgeon James Yonge met William Temple at Farnham in 1686, it appeared Temple had not conquered 'his own passions'[89] and achieved tranquillity of mind, 'Here I saw that learned and ingenious gentleman, Sir W. Temple. He is a black, sour fac'd man ... '[90]

87 'To the Reader by J.W.', in Muys, Jan (1686), *A rational practice of chyrurgery; or, Chyrurgical observations resolved according to the solid fundamentals of true philosophy ... In five decades*, London. Muys was a doctor in Arnhem. J. W. was the translator of the work.

88 William Temple, 'Upon the Gardens of Epicurus; or of Gardening in the Year, 1685', in Shaaber, p. 330. Luis Molina (1535–1600) was a Spanish Jesuit.

89 *The Journal of James Yonge*, p. 194.

90 *Idem*.

Chapter Four

Disciplined Hands

A Chirurgeon ought to be a young, or middle-ag'd Man, of a strong, steddy, and never-trembling Hand; as ready with the left Hand as with the Right; of a piercing clear Eye; he must be of an undaunted Courage, and unmerciful; fully resolv'd to go through with the Cure he has undertaken; unmoved at the Crys of his Patient, lest he either make greater haste than is convenient, or cut less than is necessary. He must, in short do everything without the least appearing Motion or Concern at the Complaints of his Patient.[1]

... no one ever endured more anxiety and sickness before an operation, yet from the time I began to operate, all uneasiness ceased; and if I have had better success than some others, I do not impute it to more knowledge but to *the happiness of mind that was never ruffled or disconcerted, and a hand that never trembled during an operation.*[2]

Perhaps you have never, or very rarely, been under the Discipline of Anatomical Hands. I fancy if you ever were to feel the Smart of a few Experiments, you'd abate of your Zeal.[3]

In 1738 William Beckett, a surgeon to St Thomas' Hospital in London, was called in by worried parents. Their three-year-old child was suffering from the after-effects of a severe case of measles. Beckett was horrified at what he found – the child's face had turned black from gangrene. He began to slice away at the dead tissue. It was distasteful work, 'I cut away the rotten, stinking, cadaverous flesh & cauterized the rest ... .' [4] Even the jawbone had become gangrenous. It 'emitted such a foetid Synomia, that the whole Room was infected with its offensive Miasms.' Beckett dug deeper and deeper with his instruments. He finally stopped when his patient signalled that he should, 'the Child, by its Strugglings, made it appear that it affected the sensible Parts.'[5] Beckett's disgust for the operation he undertook and the pity he

---

1 Sprengell, C.J., MD (1708), *The Aphorisms of Hippocrates and the Sentences of Celsus*, London, p. 332.

2 The London surgeon William Cheselden on his success in speedily removing bladder stones in (1741), *The Anatomy of the Human Body*, London, p. 334.

3 Porter, Samuel (1715), *An Essay Upon the Duty of Physicians and Patients, The Dignity of Medicine and the Prudentials of Practice, in Two Dialogues,* London, p. 23. Porter was the son of the Bishop of Oxford and graduated from Trinity College, Oxford in 1715.

4 Beckett, William (1740), *Practical surgery illustrated and improved: being chirurgical observations with remarks, upon the most extraordinary cases, cures, and dissections, made at St. Thomas's Hospital, Southwark*, London, p. 110. Beckett (1684–1738) also published on cancers, head injuries and scrofula.

5 *Idem.*.

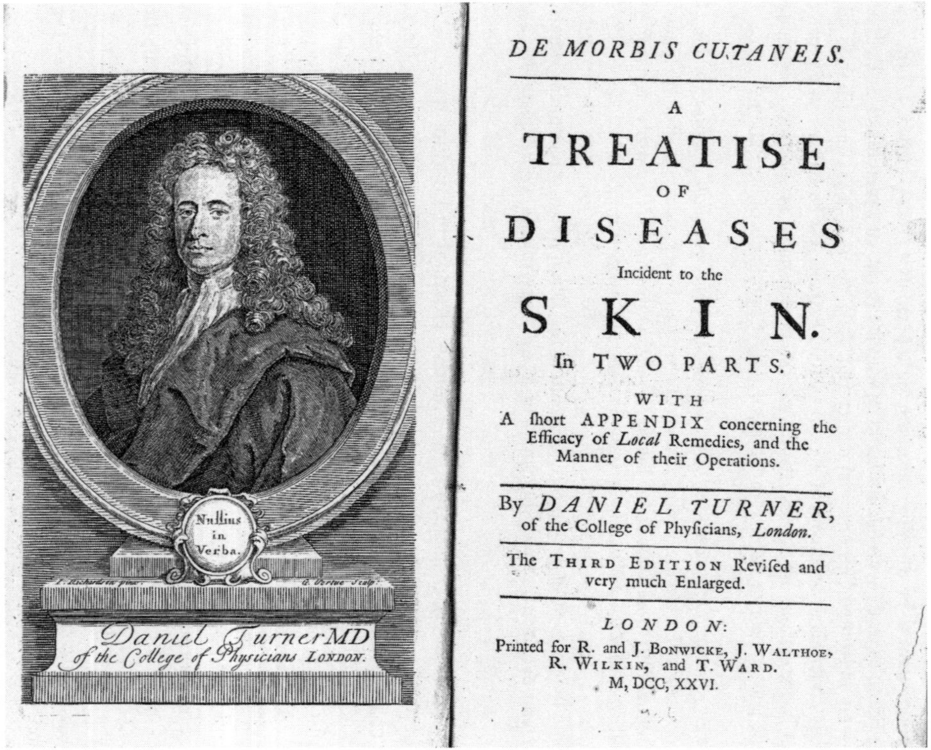

Figure 4.1 Portrait of Daniel Turner from *De Morbis Cutaneis, a Treatise of Diseases incident to the Skin*, London, 1726. By kind permission of the Clendening Library.

felt for the suffering of the child were caught in his final observation of the case, 'this miserable *object* died on the seventh Day, reckoning from the first Day the Inflammation commenced.'[6]

To work in a crowded claustrophobic room reeking of gas gangrene took a strong stomach. To cut off layer after layer of rotting flesh skilfully from a child's face took a steady hand. To judge when to persist in cutting and when to stop took a cool head. Just how did surgeons and physicians learn to tolerate working in such conditions and maintain a disciplined hand? This chapter focuses on what clinical encounters such as that of William Beckett can tell us about the passions that were aroused and suppressed by practitioners in treating patients. It examines the advice surgeons received and gave in regards to maintaining an appropriate demeanour when seeing, hearing, touching and smelling bodies in pain. What ideal traits were surgeons counselled to develop in order to possess the strength to inflict pain on their fellow men? In turn, what emotional responses were considered desirable in patients undergoing surgical treatment? How was one meant to approach surgery and what does all of this reveal about the emotional community of medical men in early eighteenth-century England?

One of the most intriguing practitioners in this context is the London surgeon and physician, Dr Daniel Turner (1667–1741).[7] While certainly not the best known of medical men in early eighteenth-century England, Turner was one of the most prolific, when it came to describing his negotiations with prospective and current patients. Indeed, Turner's emotions flash through his voluminous writings. He cajoled and tricked his patients into accepting surgical intervention and scolded and extracted confessions from them. He expressed joy when his patients recovered and sadness when illness left them with scars and disabilities. Above all, Turner sought to educate his readers in the roles and responsibilities of being a competent medical man and a good patient.[8]

As a surgeon Turner published *Apologia Chyrurgica. A Vindication of the Noble Art of Surgery* (1695). There he attacked barbers, apothecaries, quacks and anyone who practised surgery, except for trained surgeons like him. *The Present State of Chyrurgery* echoed these sentiments in 1703. Turner advertised his skill in treating skull fractures in *A remarkable case in Surgery. Wherein an account is given on an uncommon Fracture and Depression of the Skull, in a child about Six years old ...* . (1709).[9] Interestingly, William Beckett criticized Turner's identification of the cause of death and argued his treatment had prevented a cure in *Chirurgical Remarks*

6 *Idem*. Beckett's emphasis.

7 On Daniel Turner's life, see Philip K. Wilson's excellent (1999), *Surgery, Skin and Syphilis: Daniel Turner's London (1667–1741)*, Clio Medica 54, Amsterdam: Editions Rodolphi. Also, Macgee, Reginald (2003), 'Writings of Daniel Turner and his views on the practice of surgery', *ANZ. Journal of Surgery*, 73, pp. 438–42.

8 Wilson drew attention to the pedagogical aspect of Turner's writing in (1992), 'Acquiring surgical know-how: Occupational and lay instruction in early eighteenth-century London', in Porter, Roy (ed.), *The Popularisation of Medicine 1650–1850*, New York: Routledge, pp. 42–71, esp. pp. 51–2.

9 This appeared as a pamphlet with a commissioned engraving of the child's skull at autopsy. The case was later added in an abridged form to Turner's *Art of Surgery*.

Occasioned by the Death of a CHILD, whose Case was printed in that Year by Daniel Turner, surgeon, London, 1709. Turner's next work, *De Morbis Cutaneis, a Treatise of Diseases incident to the Skin* (1714), was the first book by an English author dedicated solely to skin diseases. He first considered leprosy, herpes, the itch and smallpox that 'arose inwardly' but manifested themselves externally. In Part II of the book, Turner discussed 'diseases or accidents of an outward origin', which included syphilis, burns and bites. This long treatise of 212 cases was followed by *Syphilis* (1717), *The Art of Surgery* (1721), *A Discourse concerning Fevers* (1727) and *A Discourse on Gleets* (1729).

In 1711 Turner was discharged from the Barber-Surgeons' Company and was examined and admitted as a Licentiate of the Royal College of Physicians. Twelve years later Turner shipped a parcel of 25 books to Yale College in New Haven, America. In return for the donation he requested that he be considered for an honourary Doctor of Medicine degree. In 1724 Turner received the medical degree, the first ever issued from colonial America. As Wilson records, not all were impressed by this degree. The censors of the College of Physicians refused to ratify it and some contemporaries 'jested that his M.D. more truthfully represented a *multum donavit* than a learned title.'[10]

In later life as a gentleman-physician, Turner developed a fashionable interest in antiquarian topics. He also attacked the wealthy quack Joshua Ward.[11] Like John Ward, Turner was a High Church Anglican who saw similarities between the wild ideas of medical and religious enthusiasts. He blamed the success of quacks in obtaining leave to treat bodies or save souls on the gullibility of the public. Passionate about the passions until the end of his life, Turner sparred in print with the physician James Blondel over the occurrence of maternal impressions upon the unborn child.[12] Imagination acted like the passions for Turner – it could cause emotional and physical effects. Blondel agreed that the imagination could cause the former but never the latter. Physical markings on babies resembling fruit, vegetables, fish or animals did not result from a pregnant woman craving strawberries or being frightened by a dog.[13] Turner's ambitions to silence the quacks, establish himself as an erudite and genteel medical man and to pronounce on the burning medical issues of the day, all reflect and helped form the emotional community of medical men in Enlightenment London.

10 Wilson, *Surgery, Skin and Syphilis*, p. 206.

11 Turner, Daniel (1733), *The Ancient Physician's Legacy impartially surveyed*, (1735), *The Drop and Pill of Mr. Ward considered*, and (1736), *Aphrodisiacus, a summary of the Ancient Writers on the Venereal Disease*.

12 Turner, Daniel, *'Spots and Marks'* appended to (1714), *De Morbis Cutaneis, a Treatise of Diseases incident to the Skin*, (1729), *An Answer to a pamphlet on the Power of the Imagination in Pregnant Women*, and (1730), *The Force of the Mother's Imagination upon her Foetus in Utero*. See Chapter Six of Wilson, *Surgery, Skin and Syphilis*, for a full discussion of the debate. Little is known of Blondel (1665/6–1734) except that he may have been born in Paris, was a Huguenot and received an MD from Leiden in 1692.

13 Wilson, *Surgery, Skin and Syphilis*, p. 33.

Advice for the surgeon

Roy Porter, in particular, has painted a vivid portrait of the unregulated and cut-throat eighteenth-century medical marketplace where advertised cures abounded, and licensed medical practitioners needed to fashion themselves to gain the respect of patients and their 'friends' at the bedside.[14] Engaged in a never-ending battle for the privilege of treating the bodies of patients with barbers, mountebanks, bonesetters, doctoresses and piss-prophets (not to mention other surgeons and physicians), medical men had to indulge in 'boundary maintenance', as Mary Fissell has termed it, in order to discredit their rivals.[15]

The image of Georgian medical practitioners as being beholden to their patients has been highlighted, with medicine being viewed as a commodity to be bought and sold within 'a burgeoning free-market economy, [where] medicine tacitly espoused the principles of Adam Smith, a sort of competitive individualism.'[16] This analysis has been balanced by accounts of the complex negotiations which often took place between patient and doctor over the subjective process of making a diagnosis and agreeing on a treatment.[17] While practitioners were at the mercy of market forces, they did not necessarily bow to their patients' behests. Surgery, in particular, started to rise in prestige in the early eighteenth century. As Joan Lane has detailed, the 'increased life expectancy of the eighteenth-century population and the coming of new therapies available to wealthy patients all enhanced the surgeon's status, his rise in society reflected in larger premiums and the recruitment of apprentices from gentry, mercantile and clerical homes by the 1720s.'[18]

One could train in surgery in several ways. Most common was through apprenticeship, and this was Turner's path. In 1684 he was apprenticed at age 16 to the surgeon Charles Bateman in London. Two years later Turner was 'turned over' to another surgeon, Thomas Lichfield, who was Master of the Barber-Surgeons'

---

14 There are too many works to cite. See, for example, Porter, Roy (2000), *Quacks: Fakers and Charlatans in English Medicine*, London: Tempus, and Porter, Dorothy and Porter, Roy, (1989), *Patient's Progress: Doctors and Doctoring in Eighteenth-Century England*, Stanford: Stanford University Press.

15 Fissell, Mary (1991), *Patients, Power and the Poor in Eighteenth-Century Bristol,* Cambridge and New York: Cambridge University Press, p. 155.

16 Porter, Roy (1995), 'The Eighteenth Century', in Conrad, Neve, Nutton, Porter and Wear (eds), *The Western Medical Tradition: 800 B.C. to A.D. 1800*, Cambridge: and New York: Cambridge University Press, p. 450.

17 See Duden, Barbara (1991), *The Woman Beneath the Skin. A Doctor's Patients in Eighteenth Century Germany*, trans. by Thomas Dunlap, Cambridge, MA: Harvard University Press.

18 For what little is known of surgical apprenticeships from this period see Lane, Joan (1996), *Apprenticeship in England, 1600–1914*, London: University College London Press Limited, pp. 131–3, (1988), 'Provincial Medical Apprentices and Masters in Early Modern England', *Eighteenth Century Life*, 12 (3), pp. 14–27, (2001), Lane, Joan *A Social History of Medicine: Health, healing and disease in England, 1750–1950*, London: Routledge, pp. 12–13, and Dingwall, Helen M. (1995), *Physicians, Surgeons and Apothecaries: Medicine in Seventeenth Century Edinburgh*, Edinburgh: Tuckwell Press, pp. 70–98. Quotation from Lane, *Apprenticeship*, p.131.

Company. In 1691 Turner was admitted into the freedom of the Company, but, for unknown reasons, did not take his exam until 1699 or 1700. What we do know is that Turner was an avid dissector. By age 22 and the end of his apprenticeship, he was confidently dissecting, including the body of 'A.M.,' a 30-year-old maid who had died of ascites.[19] Like many surgeons, Turner marketed his expertise in anatomy. In *The Art of Surgery* (1722) he wrote that he had devoted as 'much trouble' to each dissection and opened every corpse 'as formally as if [it were a] ... live subject'.[20] Perhaps not all his patients would have found comfort in knowing this.

Learning to become a surgeon involved mastering many skills. As Stefan Hirschauer has observed of modern surgery:

> ... the practice of operating appears to be a versatile craft. It resembles building or carpentry in the way bones are sawed, drilled, chiselled and screwed together; tailoring, where skin and tissue of different consistency are cut apart and sewn together; the work of sailors, when various knots are tied; and a butcher's trade, when muscles and innards are carved up.[21]

Pre-modern surgery required another skill, that of dispassion, when it came to inflicting pain in an attempt to heal or save the patient through cutting, blistering or amputating. How were future medical men prepared for this? What follows is twofold: a description of advice that was tendered to Enlightenment surgeons and some of their emotional reactions to operating on patients.

In 1697 an Irish medical student, Patrick Mitchell (*c.*1671–1750), attended a series of lectures in anatomy and surgery in Paris given by Monsieur Joseph Guichard Duverney (1648–1730), the Professor of Anatomy at the Jardin du Roi.[22] Mitchell's decision to pay for public courses abroad to supplement, or even replace, a traditional surgical apprenticeship was not unusual in this era.[23] Paris was a popular choice and

---

19 Biographical data has been taken from Wilson's book and (1992), 'Surgeon "turned" Physician: The Career and Writings of Daniel Turner 1667–1741', doctoral thesis, University College London, p. 42.

20 Turner, Daniel, *The Art of Surgery*, London, 1721, 1, p .272. Also see Wilson, 'Surgeon', pp. 44–5.

21 Hirschauer, Stefan (1991), 'The Manufacture of Bodies in Surgery', *Social Studies of Science*, 21, pp. 279–319, quotation from p. 300.

22 I have been able to discover only a few facts relating to Mitchell's subsequent career. From 1712–13 he was President of King and Queen's College of Physicians in Ireland. His uncle had been President from 1681–87 and was again in 1690, see Widess, J.D.H. (1963), *History of the Royal College of Ireland*, Edinburgh: Livingstone Ltd., pp. 239–42. On anatomical and surgical instruction in pre-Revolutionary Paris see Gelfand, Toby (March–April 1972), 'The "Paris Manner" of Dissection: Student Anatomical Dissection in Early Eighteenth Century Paris', *Bulletin of the History of Medicine*, 46 (2), pp. 99–130. Also, Brockliss, Laurence and Jones, Colin (1997), *The Medical World of Early Modern France*, Oxford: Clarendon Press.

23 See Lawrence, Susan (1995), 'Anatomy and Address: Creating Medical Gentlemen in Eighteenth-Century London', in *The History of Medical Education in Britain*, Nutton, Vivian and Porter, Roy (eds), Amsterdam: Rodolphi Press, pp.199–228, and *Charitable Knowledge.* Also Lawrence, Christopher (1988), 'Alexander Monro *Primus* and the Edinburgh Manner of

Duverney was one of the most respected and prestigious lecturers.[24] As many as 140 foreigners attended Duverney's lectures every year. Twenty bodies were dissected during Duverney's three-month long surgery course and 'the records of the Hôtel Dieu contain repeated complaints about Duverney's illegal purchasing of cadavers from the gravedigger of the hospital cemetery ... .'[25]

In 1698 the London physician Martin Lister, (1638–1712) recounted what he saw when he dropped in on Duverney. Lister was shown up the stairs by a young man who promptly fled back down, probably to vomit from the sights and smells he had encountered in the room:

> I was to see Monsieur *Verney* at his Apartment at the upper-end of the Royal Physick-Garden; but missing my Visit, went up with a young Gentleman of my Lord Ambassador's Retinue, to see Mr. Bennis, who was in the Dissecting Room, working by himself upon a dead Body, with its breast open and Belly gutted: There were very odd things to be seen in the Room. My Companion, it being Morning, and his Senses very quick and vigorous, was strangely surprized and offended; and retired down the Stairs much faster than he came up.[26]

Lister was affected by what he saw and felt compelled to explain why gentlemen like him would choose to work with corpses and body parts, which he referred to as 'discouraging Objects':

> And indeed, a private Anatomy Room is to one not accustomed to this kind of Manufacture, very irksome if not frightful: Here a Basket of Dissecting Instruments, as Knives, Saws, &c. and there a Form with a Thigh and Leg flayed, and the Muscles parted asunder: on another Form an Arm served after the same manner: Here a Trey full of Bits of Flesh, for the more minute discovery of the Veins and Nerves; and every where such discouraging Objects. So, as if Reason and the Good of Mankind, did not put Men upon this Study, it could not be endured: for Instinct and nature most certainly abhors the Employment.[27]

Anatomy', *Bulletin of the History of Medicine*, 62, pp. 193–214, particularly pp.195–6 and the training of Monro in Edinburgh, Paris and London.

24 Joseph Guichard Duverney (1648–1730) was Professor of Anatomy at the Jardin du Roi from 1682–1725 and Professor of Surgery and Medicine at the University of Avignon. See (1939), *Index biographique des membres et correspondants de l'academie des sciences de 1666 à 1939,* Paris: Etudes Decouverte, The *Oeuvres Anatomiques de M. Duverney*, were published in Paris in 1741.

25 Gelfand, p. 106.

26 (1967), *A Journey to Paris In the Year 1698 by Martin Lister*, Stearns, Raymond Phineas (ed.), Bloomington: University of Illinois Press, p. 66. Bennis was an English pupil of Duverney's. Lister was MD by diploma from Oxford in 1684, a member of the Royal College of Physicians and Physician in ordinary to Queen Anne. His book was immediately satirized by William King, *A Journey to London In the Year, 1698 After the Ingenuous Method of that made by Dr. Martin Lyster to Paris, in the same year &c. Written originally in French, By Monsieur Sorbiére, and Newly Translated into English*, London. Samuel Sorbiére (1615–70) was a French physician and literary hack according to Stearns. I thank Andrew Cunningham for drawing my attention to this passage.

27 *Idem.*

Reason and a godly heart, the foundations of Christian stoicism, were required to overcome the repulsion of dissecting.

Patrick Mitchell recorded in his lecture notes that Duverney began his surgery lectures with the three things necessary for making a good surgeon:

> 1. Anatomy is the foundation, of all surgery, being a guide, which gives light, into the situation, texture and diameter of the parts, e.g. in a hernia which is caused by an impulsion of the gutts ... and when a flux of blood happens, from the epigastrick arterys we know how to stopp besides its by anatomy, that we observe that part which is most necessary, and so in this distemper sometimes we sacrifys the stones to preserve the gutts.[28]

Duverney continued with an equally down-to-earth paraphrase of the Hippocratic advice of 'first do no harm':

> 2. for the second, if you have no regard to the strength of your patient, you loose your labour and reputation also, besides nothing is to attempted, till other means prove ineffectual.[29]

William Beckett combined both these pieces of advice in his treatment of the child with measles – he cut away at the face while keeping a tight eye on the strength of his patient.

Duverney finally counselled his audience that learning surgery was a manual and visual skill, and books were poor substitutes for practising anatomy:

> 3. ... the third will appear very necessary when you consider that nothing can be done without it; for the better performing of them, if you must have the rules of operating this you attain to either by reading books, or by practicing or seeing practice, reading gives, but very weak ideas of things, so you see, that people attain no more knowledge in 3 month by seeing, than in 3 years by reading ... .[30]

In stressing the necessity to 'see', 'cut' and 'practise' on the body, Duverney focused upon the two locations from which ideas regarding the body came – the eyes and the hands.[31] As he noted, books only gave 'very weak ideas'. Visually inspecting and cutting upon the body gave very strong ideas. These ideas however were not just limited to learning anatomic structures or where to cut with safety, ideas also arose in the mind of the medical man as they performed these tasks. This could result in a wavering eye and a trembling hand – not desirable traits in any surgeon. As discussed in the introduction to the book, Celsus' list of the ideal traits a surgeon should cultivate were found in many early modern medical texts.[32] According to C.J. Sprengell (1708) a surgeon was supposed to be:

28 Mitchell, Patrick (1697–98), *Lecture Notes taken in Paris mainly from the Lectures of Joseph Guichard Duverney at the Jardin du Roi from 1697–8*, Wellcome Library, MS, 6, f. 134.

29 Ibid, f. 137.

30 *Idem.*

31 In surgical training today, *see one, do one, teach one* is still quoted as the way to learn an operation.

32 For example Guy de Chauliac, famously called for 'a Lion's heart, *a Lady's hand* and a Hawk's eye'. James Yonge poked fun at clumsy surgeons in (1679) *Currus Triumphalis*,

> ... of a strong, steddy, and never-trembling Hand; as ready with the left Hand as with the Right; of a piercing clear Eye; he must be of an undaunted Courage, and unmerciful; fully resolv'd to go through with the Cure he has undertaken; unmoved at the Crys of his Patient, lest he either make greater haste than is convenient, or cut less than is necessary. He must, in short do everything without the least appearing Motion or Concern at the Complaints of his Patient.[33]

A major part of becoming a competent surgeon was learning how to discipline the imagination and so confidently wield the hand that held the knife. The question was, how was one supposed to achieve this state of dispassion? Medical texts were largely silent on this topic. Duverney, however, was not and proffered the following:

> ... by seeing and practising [on dead bodies], we accustome our selves to the bad smell of ulcers etc we loose foolish tenderness, so we can hear them cry, with out any disorder, see hemorrhages, and other accidents, after the same manner; in order to the better performing of operations, it is necessary to work on dead bodys ... .[34]

Cadavers did not cry out or gush with blood when cut.[35] This was good, as was the fact that they stank and this would prepare students for the smells they would encounter in the living – Harvey's liver abscesses or Duverney's bad ulcers. In a sense, Patrick Mitchell and his peers were being reassured by Duverney. It was normal to be foolishly tender at first when it came to cutting on a body. But here was the place where they could practise and learn to join the emotional community of medical men who could operate 'without the least appearing Motion or Concern at the Complaints of his Patient.'[36] *Appearing* calm and in control was the key to a successful surgery. Dispassion was not the same as being inhumane. As Duverney advised and William Beckett practised, the surgeon must not lose sight of the patient but continue to gauge their strength, resolve and level of pain during surgery.

Despite feelings to the contrary –'The common opinion is, that Chirurgions desire nothing more than cutting and hacking, and their Joy is at the highest pitch, when with the cutting Instruments in their Hands, they have a glut of hacking Work.'[37] – learning and maintaining humane dispassion in surgery was not easy.[38]

London, who had *'Lions paws* as well as hearts', The Introduction.

33 Sprengell, p. 332.

34 Mitchell, ff. 134–48. 'Observations taken out of a course of Cheirurgery begunn under the learned Du Verney January the 10. Anno. 1698', f. 141.

35 The fear of seeing blood is a common phobia and one that William Hunter, the subject of the next chapter, suffered from.

36 Sprengell, p. 332.

37 (1710), *Course of Chirurgical Operations, Demonstrated in the Royal Gardens at Paris by M. Dionis*, London. On the flyleaf is written, Ex Libris Jacobi Atkinson, June 20th 1727 Chirurgis, Lond: Pierre Dionis held public dissections at the Jardin du Roi between 1672 and 1680.

38 See, Lawrence, Christopher and Shapin, Steven, *Science Incarnate, Historical Embodiments of Natural Knowledge*, Chicago: University of Chicago Press ,and Wear, Andrew (2000), *Knowledge and practice in English Medicine, 1550–1680*, Cambridge and New York: Cambridge University Press.

William Cheselden (1688–1752) was a colleague of William Beckett's at St Thomas' Hospital and experienced an apprenticeship similar to Daniel Turner. Cheselden performed thousands of operations in his lifetime and made his fortune from being a speedy lithotomist. He was apprenticed at 15 to the London surgeon James Ferne and became a member of the Barber-Surgeons' Company in 1711. Two years later Cheselden had *The Anatomy of the Human Body* published. This was a manual for his students on basic operative surgery and proved to be very popular, going through 13 London editions between 1713 and 1792. In 1718 Cheselden became the principal surgeon at St Thomas' Hospital and in 1724 and 1733 respectively, he was appointed surgeon for the stone at the Westminster Infirmary and at St George's Hospital. In 1737 he was named resident surgeon at the Royal Hospital of Chelsea. William Cheselden also ran one of the earliest and most lucrative private anatomy schools in London and lectured four times a year for 20 years at St Thomas'. In 1738 he proudly published statistics demonstrating his success in lateral lithotomy, which he performed in under 30 seconds. Chesleden's data showed that of 213 patients at St Thomas' he cut for the bladder stone, only 20 died. But such success had come at a price:

> ... if I have any reputation in this way, I have earned it dearly, for *no one ever endured more anxiety and sickness before an operation, yet from the time I began to operate, all uneasiness ceased*; and if I have had better success than some others, I do not impute it to more knowledge but to *the happiness of mind that was never ruffled or disconcerted, and a hand that never trembled during an operation.*[39]

In 1730 an unruffled William Cheselden was painted by an artist in the circle of Charles Phipps, in the midst of dissecting in front of six spectators.[40] (Please see the front cover of the book). The scene is set (most probably) in one of the private anatomy rooms below the Anatomy Theatre at the Barber-Surgeons' Hall in London.

---

39 Cheselden, p. 334. Drewry Ottley, in (1835), *The Life of John Hunter*, London, refers to a famous story about Cheselden: 'Moraud relates an anecdote of a French surgeon, who, on visiting the hospital, expressed great surprise at witnessing such an evidence of weakness, as he considered it, on the part of so famous a surgeon: after the operation was over, the visitor was invited by Cheselden to accompany him to the fencing school, whither he was going to see a sparring match; but here the tables were completely turned, for no sooner did the contest begin, than the stranger turned pale at the sight, and was obliged speedily to betake himself to the open air.' Ottley adds 'Such feelings, in a less marked degree perhaps, are far more commonly experienced than is generally supposed, by the very best surgeons previously to undertaking operations of importance.' p. 9. I have not been able to verify this story and it may reflect Victorian notions of heroic surgeons rather than Enlightenment ones. See Stanley, Peter (2003), *For Fear of Pain: British Surgery, 1790–1850*, Amsterdam and New York: Rodopi.

40 Missen and Hill identify the location shown in the portrait in 'The Anatomy Theatre', see Burn (ed.), (2000) *The Company of Barbers and Surgeons*, London: The Worshipful Company of Barbers, pp. 111–28, especially pp.121–2. Beneath the theatre, the 'inventory (of 1728) lists an anatomy chest to hold instruments, a table for dissection, a hatch for the theatre door in the closets, two drawers, two planks to stand on, a pewter cistern and leaden laver (basin or sink) in the lower theatre.'

As in Padua, it appears as if small teaching groups and private dissections took place in the Lower Theatre.

The centrepiece of the painting is Chesleden's slim, white and ladylike hand. It holds a dissecting blade over the body of a naked man already split open from mid sternum to navel. Chesleden's audience appears contemplative rather than actively interested in the dissection. They largely focus upon each other or are lost in reverie while staring at Cheselden's perfect hand. As if to stress further the manual nature of surgery, the hands of three of the men also point towards the body. An open text lies disregarded in the foreground and six knives rest on the table. Skeletons are glimpsed hazily in the background, but the artist has chosen to portray the private and mundane nature of dissection for Cheselden and his admirers, rather than any religious significance.

The picture has been described as amateurish. Yet the naivety captures the importance of the hand in surgery for revealing the sight and, therefore, understanding the structures in the body. Chesleden equated seeing with knowing in his hugely popular anatomy text for students:

> In describing of the parts, I have pretty much neglected the Minutiae in ANATOMY: Nor have I been very particular about those Things which cannot be understood without being seen, and being seen need little description.[41]

Surgeons relied on cutting to reveal knowledge. Dissecting the dead was easy as Duverney pointed out for they did not scream or bleed. Cheselden's subject lays peacefully on the table. But cutting on the living was another matter. It took physical and emotional skills. Surgeons were told that cutting on the dead would prepare them for cutting on the living. But what of the patients? What advice if any, were they given on how they were supposed to behave during operations? How did the ideal and the real measure up, and what does all of this tell us about the emotional community of medical men in early eighteenth-century England?

Advice for the patient

The verbose Daniel Turner naturally had advice for his patients. He called for them to confide in him, obey his instructions and remain stoic in the knowledge that he had their best interests at heart:

> I wish that every Patient would make choice of such an honest and able Professor of this Art as they might reasonably confide in, and then wholly, under the Supreme Power, submit themselves (without dictating their own erroneous Sentiments) to his management. I would have them banish all those childish and fearful Apprehensions of his supposed Cruelty, and remain stedfast, in a firm belief, that he will act no otherwise by them than himself, if under such circumstances; or, that what he does is purely design'd for their recovery and wellbeing.[42]

---

41 Cheselden, Preface, p. 5.

42 Turner, Daniel (1695), *Apologia Chyrurgica Or A Vindication of the Noble Art of Surgery*, London, p. 121.

Several themes are present here: the necessity of patients to submit to the authority of a good surgeon as a child should to a good father, the rationality of the medical practitioner as opposed to the erroneous sentimentality of the patient, and the image of the surgeon as benevolent and knowledgeable and a person in which the patient must blindly place faith.

This was Turner at the beginning of his career in 1693. He would become 'one of the most outspoken London authors on venereal disease' and treat hundreds with symptoms of the French disease.[43] Turner has even been credited with introducing the condom to Londoners in his *Syphilis, A Practical Dissertation of Venereal Disease*, (1717). Surgeons earned a lot of income and fame from treating poxed patients, and in one sense it was easy work – they never lacked for patients given the high rates of sexually transmitted diseases in Georgian society. A quarter to a third of the population of London is estimated to have had the pox.[44] But treating the venereally diseased was difficult work for the surgeon. As Kevin Siena states, 'Being labelled "foul" brought with it a range of ramifications that went well beyond dispensing mercury. At stake were important issues of privacy and reputation, which, if damaged, could bring serious economic results.'[45] Preserving their reputations led to arguments, denials and lies:

> In their attempts to preserve their privacy, venereal patients initially benefited from the early modern medical exchange, a process of negotiation between doctor and patient in which the patient played an active role in constructing their own diagnosis. In a word, patients were given an important voice within the medical exchange in the period up to the mid-eighteenth century. Venereal patients took advantage of that opportunity and actively contested their diagnosis. Some resisted being labeled 'foul.' Others used the chance to obscure or rewrite sexual history.[46]

Daniel Turner found all of this to be true and it aroused his passions and tested his benevolence towards patients.

In 1732 Turner described cases of pox he had diagnosed and treated for 30 years in the voluminous *Syphilis: A Practical Dissertation on the Venereal Disease in Two Parts*.[47] The cases are not dated and most of them suggest that he had a difficult time getting patients to confide, obey and be as stoic as possible. Turner's patience and stoicism was often challenged:

> History VI. A very precise and exact Gentleman, pretending to a more than ordinary strict Profession, complained of great Pain in his Members, which with some Difficulty I was

43 Wilson, Philip K. (1999), *Surgery, Skin and Syphilis: Daniel Turner's London (1667–1741)*, Clio Medica, 54, Amsterdam: Editions Rodolphi, p. 150.

44 Siena, Kevin (2004), *Venereal Disease, Hospitals and the Urban Poor*, Rochester: University of Rochester Press, p. 10.

45 Ibid, p. 8.

46 Ibid., p. 13.

47 It is over 600 pages long.

> admitted to see; and found one of the *Testes* much tumefied, which he said was occasioned by his lying cross-legg'd in his Sleep.[48]

Turner did not fall for the story of a swollen testicle being caused by sleeping with crossed legs. But until he could extract the truth from the patient he went along with it. He finally called in another surgeon, Mr Richard Blundell – or perhaps the patient's friends requested another opinion – after the patient got no better from treating his swelling as a simple bruise. 'Together taking a View' the two surgeons thought that the enlarged testicle might be seminal retention from celibacy or most likely, 'notwithstanding his Character, it might be venereal'. They continued to purge the patient and Turner carefully observed his demeanour, 'In the Morning I found him much easier, yet perpetually sighing, which encreased my Suspicion of the real Cause.'[49] Turner then began to purge the gentleman aggressively and watched with satisfaction as his testicle started to empty. He finally found an opportunity to force the patient to confide – in a characteristically graphic and physical fashion. Turner pointed out to the man of the cloth that the drainage on the bed sheets looked like that from pox. He then grabbed hold of the patient's dripping penis before he could hide it from him:

> ... coming one Morning ... I observed his Linen stained with a Running, which I shewed him; at the same time taking hold of the *Penis*, that he had before used very industriously to conceal, I found the like Matter issuing therefrom, which I was very glad to see ... .[50]

The game was up. Turner comforted his patient. Now he knew what was really wrong with him, he could cure him. The patient broke down, cried and begged Turner to be careful of his 'Reputation which was considerable among his Party, and I promis'd him that I would. After this we went on more chearfully ... .'[51]

Turner's fearful gentleman, perhaps a vicar, was considered lucky by Turner and Blundell. They believed he was suffering most likely from a local clap and not the more generalized pox that developed if the clap was not treated. A clap involved a sore, pain on urination and a yellow discharge or 'gonorrhoea'. If not eradicated, it moved inward to attack organs and eventually the entire body.[52] The patient experienced excruciating bone pain and oozing skin eruptions; inflamed genital regions swelled and became gangrenous.[53] The standard treatment was mercury – given orally, topically or through fumigation. Mercury is a sudorific and causes copious sweating and drooling. Saliva was carefully measured in pints as evidence of the venereal poison leaving the body. The treatment was toxic and prolonged and caused terrible side effects. Patients had abdominal pain, nausea, lost their teeth, had

48 Turner, Daniel (1732), *Syphilis: A Practical Dissertation on the Venereal Disease, in Two Parts,* London, p. 245.

49 Ibid., p. 245.

50 Ibid., p. 246.

51 *Idem.*

52 Siena, p. 17.

53 Ibid., pp. 17–20.

bleeding gums and their uvula rotted.[54] Their breath stank and they lost their voices. This is the treatment Turner saved his patient from. These were not easy patients to diagnose or treat in terms of getting them to admit their sexual history, and Turner expressed his frustration in case after case. Called in to see a pregnant gentlewoman with a sore throat, he found a 'sordid Ulcer on the Base of the *Uvula* ... Upon this, in private, I acquainted the Husband, who I found was too conscious of Liberties he had taken, to need many Arguments upon that Subject ... .'[55] The stern father figure that is seen in so many of Turner's and other surgeons' histories is well caught here.[56] The husband begged Turner to return the woman's voice – as loss of voice was a cardinal and public sign of the pox. The woman's reaction to the treatment is not recorded but she must have known from the mercury being prescribed that her sore throat resulted from being poxed.

In 1714 Turner published the first work in English concerning skin diseases. Entitled *De Morbis Cutaneis*, the author carefully described himself as a *former* member of the Barber-Surgeons' Company, *now* a Licentiate of the College of Physicians of London. However, the treatment of skin diseases, including syphilis, was traditionally the work of a surgeon. Turner illustrated his various chapters upon 'Fancy-Marks' (Birth Marks), burns, bruises, insect bites and of the 'natural passages imperforate' (blocked orifices) with a selection of his own cases where he revealed the risks he took (in hindsight) when treating patients.[57]

Called in merely to stop the bleeding from a raspberry birthmark near a gentlewoman's eyebrow, Turner talked her into having this 'whole Fungus removed' despite the woman superstitiously, according to Turner, 'fancying it both sinful and fruitless to attempt removing a Mark of God Almighty's sending.' Turner explained that his expertise in anatomy ensured a good result. 'Incouraging her with great Hopes of Success', he then vividly described how he had to cut out the seedy tainted skin down to the very bone.[58] Pleased with his handiwork, Turner left the patient to recuperate. However he was undermined by one of the patient's friends and grumpily recounted:

> When some officious Person in my absence, telling her that her Skull lay bare, and that it went down to her Brain, she was much displeas'd that I had undertaken it.[59]

Upon his return to the patient's bedside, Turner rushed to repair the damage done by the woman's friend. He confidently reassured his patient that she had done the right thing and that by surrendering to his arguments she had even ensured that the raspberry mark would never grow back. But Turner revealed his worries regarding the excision to his readers:

---

54 Ibid., p. 23.

55 Turner, *Syphilis*, p. 258.

56 See for example, *The Diary of James Yonge* and the works of James Cooke.

57 Of 212 case histories, 141 were from ancient or contemporary writers and 71 from his patients.

58 Turner, Daniel (1714), *De Morbis Cutaneis*, London, p. 125.

59 *Idem.*

> Had I apprehended it so deeply rooted, I might not probably have been so very forward in the Undertaking, unless I had been solicited thereto by the Patient: But discovering after how it was, I was resolv'd to follow it even down to the Cranium ... rather than leave it to sprout anew, to the Patient's farther Inconvenience and my own Discredit.[60]

A crucial part of the doctor-patient interaction was to establish the indebtedness of the latter to the former by having the patient solicit the skills of the doctor rather than vice versa. Turner appeared to have recognized from this incident that he had come dangerously close to acting like a quack by boasting of his abilities before making a careful anatomical examination of the patient. In essence, Turner had been so preoccupied with overcoming the patient's fears that he had failed to exercise sufficient dispassion in treatment or prognosis.

The choice of words in this clinical encounter alone is revealing of the hard work it took for Turner to maintain emotional control over himself, the patient and her friends. Turner 'convinced', 'prevailed', 'encouraged', 'comforted' and 'assured' the patient. She 'complied'. Roy Porter has cautioned that:

> Faculty-talk and quackspeak need to be treated symmetrically. Both orthodox and irregular medicine generated their own linguistic sub-cultures, whose vocabulary, tones and speech mannerisms, though somewhat distinct, played similar socially and even therapeutically active roles.'[61]

Like the quacks he despised, Turner tried to inspire confidence – 'Incouraging her with great Hopes of Success'. At times he harangued his patients, at other times he threatened them, and sometimes he made fun of them.

Turner responded to a call for treatment of an inflamed 'Labia pudendi' in a young woman with prescriptions by post and then, when these proved inadequate, a personal visit. He found, 'all the outsides of the Labia from the Pubes quite down to the Perinaeum ... black and fetid' and quickly diagnosed gonorrhoea on account of 'the wanton use she had made of her parts'.[62] Like William Beckett, Turner set to and removed all the dead tissue, but unlike Beckett he used caustics and not a knife. He left a supply of dressings for the young woman to apply daily to keep the labia moist and separated. However the patient was not compliant:

> ... being perfectly easie [she] arose daily and went abroad, by which her Dressings falling into Wrinkles, were apt to slip off, and in one Night's Time ... by her Negligence, the Parts were growing fast together.[63]

Turner returned and scolded her. He took particular delight in ruthlessly extracting a future promise of obedient and chaste behaviour by threatening to leave her vagina imperforate:

---

60 Turner, *De Morbis*, p. 126.

61 Porter, Roy (1987), 'The language of quackery in England, 1660–1800', in Burke, Peter and Porter, Roy (eds), *The Social History of Language*, Cambridge and New York: Cambridge University Press, pp. 73–103, quotation from p. 76.

62 Turner, *De Morbis*, p. 242.

63 Ibid., p. 243.

> I ask'd her jestingly, if she was content, provided we took Care to secure a Passage for her Urine, to let the other part remain as it was; which (to hear what she would say) I told her could not be now parted without a great deal of Pain: She beg'd I would assist her, and divide it with as little Pain to her as possible, promising to be more careful as well as chast for the Future. I then try'd with my Probe, but that was not strong enough, being very small; but with the edge of my *Spatula* I got through, she crying out, as I told her she must expect.[64]

Turner was well aware of the pain his patients experienced; here he warned the woman as he proceeded of what she must expect from his efforts.

In another case he was obviously disturbed by the torments his patient experienced. This was a 'maiden Gentlewoman about twenty with a good face', who fell into the kitchen grate. Turner found her 'miserably burnt all over her Face' and down one breast and an arm. He 'gently' wiped off the 'Sallet Oil' with a feather that the household women had smeared her burns with, dressed the horrific wounds and left her in the care of another local surgeon, Mr William Petty.[65] The patient's pain was so severe that Turner was called in at two o'clock in the morning. He supplied the patient with:

> *Sydenham's* liquid' laudanum: I was forced to allow the *Laudanum* 15 Drops Morning and Evening, which somewhat blunted the Extreminty of the Pain, alth' one half of the Day, especially for some Hours after Dressing (tho' I used her as tenderly as 'twas possible) she lamented like a Person (as indeed she was) in the greatest Agony.[66]

Turner dwells on her pain throughout this case history. He reports that he and Richard Blundell heard her screams as they entered the house each day and he wonders at the patient's stoic fortitude, just as John Ward had wondered at Mrs Townshend's as they amputated her breast:

> ... it may be imagin'd the Pain must be in a Manner insupportable, and that the Stoical Apathy it self (were such a Thing to be found) must now buckle to humane Frailty and marke its just Complaints, which were as well moderated by the patient Submission of this young Gentlewoman (all Things consider'd) as could with any Reason be expected.[67]

In *The Art of Surgery,* first published in 1721, Turner detailed many cases where he was called in to examine women, post-partum, who were suffering from severely inflamed breasts.[68]

Turner did not mince words with patients who did not comply with his orders. He was quick to scold and intimidate one patient with a severely ulcerated breast who,

64 Ibid., p. 244.

65 Ibid., p. 270.

66 Ibid., p. 271.

67 Ibid., p. 272.

68 Turner, *The Art of Surgery,* London, 1729. There are 107 cases described in 1,096 pages. In 14 of the cases he consulted with William Petty and of the 21 patients who died Turner gained permission to dissect 7 of them.

with the help of her nurse, had removed his tent. This was a piece of lint that was inserted to keep a wound open and wick away the drainage. It was painful:

> When I came the next Morning, and was inform'd what had been done, I told her plainly, If she would not give way to what I had therby propos'd, it would be to no purpose to give farther Attendance; endeavouring once more to convince her, that until we had an Orifice, that might favour the emptying of her Breast, she might be in the same Plight, if not much worse ... half a year after … .[69]

Turner wanted compliance and obedience and attempted to achieve both by appealing to the woman's common sense. But the patient did not prove 'pliable' and Turner dispassionately resolved to leave her, rather than risk a failed cure and damage to his reputation.[70] Yet on his final visit 'espying' her breast once more, he could not resist the opportunity to plunge his probe into one of the ulcerated areas and finding the patient tolerated this procedure 'somewhat', Turner decided to grant her a second chance. He reassured her that if she would submit to him placing the tent inside the breast again for three days, he would guarantee a cure.

Yet, once again, the patient did not keep her part of the bargain. Turner's patient found 'her Courage it seems, failing, or her Pain surmounting'. She sent a messenger the next morning to Turner, stating that if he did not come and drain the breast that moment she would once again pull out the tent herself. This time Turner was ready. He entered the vacillating patient's sickroom armed with 'a large Steel-Instrument ... into which I had drawn about a dozen Needles-full of stitching Silk.'[71] He found his patient close to fainting and holding a large basin under her breast to catch the copious discharging matter:

> Hereupon, unwilling to lose this Opportunity, with my Probe, as usually, in my Hand, as if going to pass the same, whilst my Patient was thus leaning upon her Nurse's Arm with her Head, in a sort of *Deliquiium*, or *Lypothymy*, I chang'd my Probe unheeded to them both, and, concealing the Silk in my Hand, pass'd down the Steel one, and forc'd the same through with very little Complaint, having kept them ignorant of what I had done ... .[72]

A month later, he wrote, the breast was completely cured and the lady fulsome in her praises of his medical skill – if not his bedside manner.

Turner recognized, as all good surgeons did, that courage and pain are linked: one generally decreases as the other increases. Why did Turner choose to treat the patient in such a cavalier way? He mentions that she had left him once before, perhaps she had told others that he had failed to cure her then and he was determined to do so this time. Turner also was very confident he could resolve this patient's problem if he she would only let him. He could not obtain her obedience so he circumvented it. But he attempted to do this in a humane way – by hiding the instruments and not revealing his plan. This was age-old advice, found in Hippocrates and Galen as well as early modern surgical texts. It must be noted though that Turner took particular

69 Ibid., 2, p. 367.

70 *Idem*.

71 Ibid., 2, p. 368.

72 *Idem*.

pleasure in getting his patients's to obey his wishes and was prepared to put them in considerable pain to do so.

The punitive element in the work of physicians, and particularly surgeons, was well recognized in the early eighteenth century. For example, in the anonymous treatise *An Essay Upon the Duty of Physicians and Patients: The Dignity of Medicine and the Prudentials of Practice, in Two Dialogues* (1715) two imaginary patients, Mesdames Jasmilla and Olympia, bantered back and forth about the purported cruelty of the medical profession. Jasmilla began:

> Perhaps you have never, or very rarely, been under the Discipline of Anatomical Hands. I fancy if you ever were to feel the Smart of a few Experiments, you'd abate of your Zeal.[73]

To this Olympia countered:

> Incision-Knives were not made for Ceremonie. When the Rule require it, the Physitian is as much bound to torture a man into Health, as a Judge to give Sentence. For Cancers and Gangreens are as Incorrigible, as Harded'd Malefactors.[74]

Turner agreed with Olympia. In his opinion it was the duty of a respectable and learned medical man, such as himself, to treat patients whether or not they had the courage to be treated. Turner was far from being the aggressor and claimed that upon hearing the 'clamorous shrieks and Outcries of poor suffering' patients, a practitioner often became an 'almost equal Sufferer'.[75] This was evident in the case of the woman who was horribly burnt in the fire.

Turner treated children frequently and made no allowances for their tender age in his willingness to ensure compliance. In the case of a seven-year-old boy with an imperforate penis, Turner opened the passage and left a wax candle 'besmear'd with a Bit of fresh Butter' in the ductus to keep it open. But the child pulled it out during the night and 'finding some Smart in putting the Candle back again, he threw it away'. Notified by the family of this disregard of his orders, Turner replaced the candle and then threatened the boy 'by saying he should be cut again, if he play'd any more such Tricks.'[76]

Infants and children were notoriously difficult to diagnose and treat because they lacked the ability to give a rational history. Walter Harris, a physician and

---

73 Anonymous, (1715), *An Essay Upon the Duty of Physicians and Patients: The Dignity of Medicine and the Prudentials of Practice, in Two Dialogues,* London, p. 23.

74 *An Essay Upon*, p. 24. See Harley, David (1993), 'Ethics and Dispute Behaviour in the Career of Henry Bracken of Lancaster: Surgeon, Physician and Man Midwife', in Baker, Robert, Porter, Dorothy and Porter, Roy (eds), *The Codification of Medical Morality: Historical and Philosophical Studies of the Formalization of Western Medical Morality in the Eighteenth and Nineteenth Centuries*, Dordrecht: Kluwer Academic Publications, pp. 51–2, for Turner's contemporary, Henry Bracken's vexations regarding the image of surgeons as butchers.

75 Wilson, *Surgery, Skin and Syphilis*, p. 52. From Turner, *Apologia Chyrurgica*, pp. 121–2.

76 Turner, *The Art of Surgery*, 2, p. 233.

surgeon to William and Mary, published one of the first medical texts devoted to very young patients in 1693. He captured the frustration and fear medical men faced in diagnosing and treating them:

> I know in how unfrequented, and unknown a Path I am to walk, since Children, and especially sick Infants offer nothing for a clear Diagnostick, but what we can collect from their moaning Complaints, & their uncertain Idiom of frowardness [sic]; wherefore, very many Physicians of the best Vogue, have often declared to myself, what unwilling Visits they made to Sick, but especially New born Children; hoping little from these Notices for the unridling of their Maladies.[77]

Turner took great pride in instructing his audience of young medical men how to treat recalcitrant children. Unable to stop a child's neck bleeding after removing two leeches and applying pressure for an hour, Turner resorted to tricking the infant and his nurse:

> Whilst I was musing what I had best to do, I espy'd a Tobacco-Pipe in the Chimney-Corner, and put the same into the Fire, not letting the Nurse know my Intention.[78]

Turner then 'took his opportunity' to 'suddenly clapt the End of it red hot as it was upon the Bleeding-Hole.'[79] There appears to have been a tradition, prior to Turner, of stories regarding the means some surgeons took to trick their patients into a painful cure. The surgeon Alexander Reid observed of the fear on seeing the knife:

> But because some faint-hearted Patients are afraid of this Instrument, Chirurgians have devised to fasten the point of a Lancet or Knife in the midst of a peece of Coyne, to stand out as far as they would have the wound to be deep. That coyne they cover with some thin Cearecloath, to hide the edge or point, pretending that cearecloth to bee the Medicine which shall make way for the matter to issue; but when they have cunningly conveyed the Coyne upon the Apostemation, suddenly they presse it as hard as they meane to make the Incision deepe ... .[80]

There were many barriers in surgery – some were put up by the patient while others were erected by the surgeon. The 'cearecloth' (silk cloth) in Reid's account was one, and Turner's threats of further pain if you didn't behave well now was another.

Turner's professional pride was severely ruffled when he was called in to examine a gentleman who had bruised his legs by drunkenly falling out of a boat. The surgeon arrived to discover a 'Chymist' present and the patient apparently still drunk:

---

77 Harris, Walter (1693), *An Exact Enquiry into, and Cure of the Acute Diseases of Infants*, by Walter Harris, MD, Englished by W.C. M.S. With a Preface in Vindication of the Work. London. Harris argued that all childhood disorders were due to an excess of acid. The quotation is from Harris's Preface.

78 Turner, *The Art of Surgery*, 2, p. 340.

79 Ibid., 2, p. 341.

80 Reid, Alexander (1634), *A Description of the Body of Man*, London, p. 5. This was from a chapter upon the 'opening of Tumors'.

> I was somewhat startled that he should call me in to consult with a person of another Profession, and who knew Nothing of the Matter. But the Gentleman in a merry Humour told me, he had sent for me to convince me of the great Efficacy of Spirit of Wine in curing Bruises with extravasate Blood; I would only (says he) desire you with your best Art to take the Care of one Leg, and my Friend shall take the other with his Spirit of Wine.[81]

Turner 'to carry on the Frolick', agreed to the challenge explaining that, 'I thought I needed no better Opportunity of making an Experiment.' Turner dressed the appointed leg with an *Anodyne Cataplasm,* while the Chymist sprinkled the other with his spirit of wine. On returning the next morning they found the patient restless and in pain due to an inflammation developing on the leg treated by the Chymist. Naturally, Turner immediately pointed this out:

> To this they both reply'd it was usual with the Spirit to create a little Pain and Inflammation, which was owing to the Subtilty and Volatility of its alcalious Particles dissolving the Acid of the grumous Blood, but afterwards when it had rendred the same fluid, and fitted it to be return'd by the Circulation, those Symptoms went off quickly after.[82]

The surgeon responded to this convoluted explanation with an attack, not upon its medical content, but upon the method, which he found distinctly lacking:

> I told the Chymist I value'd no *Hypotheses* whose *Phaenomena* did not regularly and orderly correspond, and whose Facts (grounded upon common Experience) did not corroborate the same, not being coined in our own Imaginations and brought in, to serve a Turn.[83]

He accused the Chymist of being a quack who used his imagination rather than his reason to sell a cure. Turner departed, returning two days later with the Chymist to discover that a massive abscess now stretched from the toes to the groin on the leg treated by the Chymist:

> I askt my Brother Surgeon what he thought of it, he said he believ'd it Blood not yet return'd [to the heart]; I then askt my Patient jestingly, if he was willing to wait the Return of it, at the same time assuring him there was Matter, and that it was fit to be let out, nor ought to lye there any longer.[84]

Turner went on to drain near half a pint of pus from the abscess, and it took him another six weeks to heal the wound completely. In his duel with the Chymist over the increasingly pain-wracked body of their patient, Turner again reflected on the value coming to be placed on professional authority based on empirical experience and efficacy. The practical anatomical knowledge and social status of Turner were pitted successfully against that of the Chymist. Both men offered the patient diagnosis and prescription but only Turner could deliver 'the efficacious particulars and clever

81 Turner, *De Morbis,* p. 250.
82 Ibid., p. 251.
83 *Idem.*
84 *Idem.*

observations gathered from experience' and apply them with dispassionate eyes and hands.[85]

For ambitious medical men, such as Turner, conducting autopsies was a way to derive both personal and public satisfaction. Turner, like many others, had gained competency through first practising on the dead, and it was to the dead he returned when he wished to preserve his reputation. One of his most detailed case histories involves the dissection of a six-year-old boy from Moorfields who was hit in the head by a 'catstick'. Turner recounted that 'On the 24th of February, 1708–9, I was called in much haste to a Child ... taken up for dead, and continued speechless for some time.'[86] With the aid of other surgeons, including Walter Herenden, the Warden of the Company of Barber-Surgeons, Turner performed various operations on the child's skull, including taking the scalp off so the complete fracture could be viewed and trepanned twice.

Turner described each surgery in military terms as an assault on the body, as indeed it was. He 'armed' his instruments and 'redoubled his force' in using them, while the patient was described in terms of his courage as a 'soldier' and a 'champion'. When Turner removed a piece of the scalp 'my Patient never winch'd at; although he told his Nurse the Day before, he thought, at his first cutting, we would not leave him, until we had taken off all the Flesh from that side of his Head.'[87]

The need for a steady hand is nicely demonstrated in Turner's description of the operations. He draws on the head, cuts the scalp to expose the fracture, and his assistant inserts his fingers under the bone to estimate the size of the injury:

> I began to draw a semicircular Line on the outside of the Depression, as a direction for my Knife ... . Then, whilst Mr. *Blundel* kept the Head steady, I cut through my half Circle to the *Cranium,* and found I was just beyond the edge of the fractur'd Bone; but, drawing my Knife upon the strait Line, it slip'd in a considerable distance from the superfices unawares; which my Assistant perceiving, I withdrew the same to make way for his Finger, by which he discover'd so great a Vacuity, that we concluded the Bones were beat through both *Meninged,* into the Substance of the Brain.[88]

After nearly three months, the skull fracture turned gangrenous and the child died, leaving Turner to wax poetic upon:

> ... this little Hero, of truly manly Courage, who had struggled under, and got through so many Difficulties, and seemed now, in vulgar Estimation, to have been well and out of danger for a long time past, at last decease, after four score and four Days.[89]

Turner then set to and dissected the child's head, taking the brain out to examine it and discreetly sewing the scalp back together:

---

85 Cook, Harold J., (January, 1994), 'Good Advice and Little Medicine', *Journal of British Studies,* 33, pp. 1–31, quotation from p. 30.

86 Turner, *The Art of Surgery*, 2, p. 223.

87 Ibid., p. 228.

88 Ibid., p. 225.

89 Ibid., p. 245.

> The Day after his Death, I took with me a small capital Saw, and a dissecting Knife, and placing the Head to my Advantage, I divided the Scalp from the Base of the Occiput, close by the Saggital Suture, to the top of the Forehead. Having thus far satisfy'd my own Curiosity, I placed the Brain where I found it, and fitting to, the divided Skull, drew over the Scalp: which stitching up, and, with the point of my Needle raising the short Hair, to cover the said Stitches, 'twas no easy matter for the nicest Surveyor, to perceive that the Brain had been taken out and inspected, or the Cranium meddled with: But this only by the by.[90]

Having privately satisfied his curiousity Turner had the case published, first as a pamphlet in 1709, *A remarkable case in Surgery. Wherein an account is given on a uncommon Fracture and Depression of the Skull, in a child about Six years old* … . It was later added to *The Art of Surgery*. He was so proud of this case that he commissioned an engraving of the skull detailing each of his many operations on its surface. The picture stood as an objective history of his manual dexterity in this ultimately fatal case.

Turner's telling of this case echoes the surgeon James Yonge's description of a four-year-old boy he cured in 1679 of two large penetrating wounds to the *Dura* and *Pia mater.* After a gate fell on him the child demonstrated the same stoic qualities that Turner's little 'champion' did in receiving treatment:

> And here I cannot forbear to celebrate the admirable, and as it were prudent, courage of this little Gentleman, more especially remarkable in three things; First, That he was very quiet and steady, scarce wincing at whatever was done; and this from a sense of its being beneficial and inevitable: as appears by the second, That when one of the By-standers (whilst I cut him) observing him mute, feared him to be a swound, and peeping into his face, ask'd him how he did, he briskly replyed, Pretty well; and, as if he had apprehended the cause of her enquiry, added, *They don't hurt me.* Thirdly, That once, on a more painful and tedious dress than ordinary, he prevented himself from crying by biting a Linnen Cloth hard in his teeth, and pulling it with both hands; A cunning way to ease himself, and be silent![91]

Yonge was engaged in a debate with a Dr W. Dirlton of Plymouth who did not believe Yonge could have cured the child because Hippocrates had declared wounds of the brain to be always mortal. Yonge countered by stating that relying on the ancients and their aphorisms could be deceptive and pointed to everyday experiences which were modifying the ancients, especially new anatomical studies:

> What is there in the Anatomy of the Brain (especially the Cortical part) as delivered to us by the hands and most renowned *Willis, Highmore,* and *Malpighius,* that can justifie your opinion?[92]

Here the process of creating medical knowledge by early modern surgeons such as Yonge and Turner can be seen, for in their very description of body parts and diseases

90 Ibid., p. 247.

91 Yonge, James (1682), *Wounds of the Brain proved Curable*, London, p. 27.

92 Ibid., p. 59.

was the emphasis of the possibility, indeed, the very desirability of performing surgery. New knowledge was delivered by the discipline of anatomical hands.

In 1727 Turner had published a work on fevers which included 'letters' on the conduct and character of a physician. *A Discourse Concerning Fevers in Two Letters To a Young Physician, Directing his Regimen for the Cure, and his Conduct to the Sick Person* advised young medical men to keep their distance from patients:

> I would never have you over familiar, at least not so as to be often at their Tables; for this in time will also make you cheap; and there are those who instead of seeing you handsomely, will be apt to place your Visits to the Account of their Civilities, and treat you rather as their *Friend* than *Physician*. Be affable with them and sociable as you will, but cautious how you dip your Finger in their Dish, or take a Bottle at their Cost.[93]

He warned future surgeons and physicians to avoid discussing politics and religion and to be sober and moral. Don't burst into 'the Chambers of the Sick, with a D___n it, what a Pulse is here? Z___s what a Urine? or with Grimace break some sorry Jest at the Bedside, as I have been Witness of.'[94] Such conversation must be shunned 'like the Plague for fear of Infection'.[95]

Having discussed conduct, Turner turned to the character to which a young medical man should aspire. First, be learned and of good judgement with an expert knowledge of anatomy and frequent dissections of *morbid bodies*; second, be confidential and don't babble about your patients's problems; third, be honest, grave and modest; fourth, be discreet and dress the part; and fifth, try to sympathize with what your patients are feeling:

> It will behove him to appear always neat in his Attire, avoiding the Extremes of the Fop and the Sloven, with a chearful Countenance, especially before the Sick; rather compassionating their Infirmities, than resenting every little Excursion which Pain and Peevishness may extort from some of them; for as Pity and Humanity are due to all Men under Affliction, so no Man shews these most excellent Endowments with a better Grace than does the Physician.[96]

Above all, learn to keep 'that becoming Distance with his Patient, as may procure to him the greater Reverence and Respect.'[97]

Based on his case histories, it is hard to recognize Turner as the model for some of this discourse. Yet his advice captures the difficulty practitioners faced in establishing their authority over patients and maintaining the appropriate distance. During his long career Turner attempted to advertise and use his superior anatomical judgement to gain access to, and establish lasting control over, his patients' bodies and emotions. To do this, he had to defeat the claims of competing practitioners to provide more efficacious and perhaps more painless cures. Next Turner had to devalue the patients' (and their friends') knowledge of their own sickness and get

93 Turner, Daniel (1739), *A Discourse Concerning Fevers*, London, p. 328.
94 *Idem*.
95 Ibid., p. 330.
96 Ibid., p. 333.
97 Ibid., p. 332.

them to confide in him. Anatomizing, in conjunction with many years of operating on patients, shaped Turner's outlook on the conduct and character required of someone who, on a daily basis, had to endure the assault of humans in pain. His many published works provide valuable insight into the emotional and moral stance an early modern medical man took towards his patients, their illnesses, the behaviour of bystanders at their bedsides and other medical practitioners.

Chapter Five

Necessary Inhumanity

> It is dissection alone that can teach us, where we may cut the living body, with freedom & dispatch; and where we may venture, with great circumspection and delicacy, and where we must not, upon any account attempt it. This informs the *head*, gives dexterity to the *hand*, and familiarises the *heart* with a sort of *necessary inhumanity*, the use of cutting instruments upon our fellow-creatures.[1]

> DISPASSION ... Freedom from mental perturbation.
> DISPASSIONATE ... Cool; calm; moderate; temperance.[2]

> Anatomy ... is to this day, and must be to the end of time, new, entertaining, useful, and inexhaustible.[3]

On 8 October 1793 James Williams, a 16-year-old medical student, wrote a letter to his sister Mary in Worcester.[4] James was a pupil of John Hunter, the renowned anatomist and surgeon.[5] In a previous letter Mary had asked her brother to describe his living quarters at the anatomy school. James replied:

---

1 Simmons, Simon Foart (1784), *Two Introductory Lectures, delivered by William Hunter, to his last course of Anatomical Lectures, at his Theatre in Windmill-Street: As they were left corrected for the Press by himself. Printed by order of the Trustees, for J. Johnson*, London, p, 62. Brock points out on pp. 40 and 60 that the manuscript was actually titled *Two Introductory Lectures by Dr. Hunter. Read at his New Theatre on the first and second day of Oct., 1767*, and includes additions and corrections added throughout the years. Simmons was an alienist who treated George III in 1803. He only had a glancing acquaintance with William Hunter.

2 Johnson, Samuel (1786), *A Dictionary of the English Language in which the words are deduced from their originals*, 8th ed., I, London. The dictionary consulted was owned by Edward Jenner and is now in the Clendening Library at the University of Kansas Medical Center. My thanks to the Rare Books Librarian, Dawn McInnis, for drawing my attention to it.

3 Simmons, p. 67.

4 Edwards, G. (1968), 'John Hunter's Last Pupil', *Annals of the Royal College of Surgeons of England*, 42, pp. 68–70. James added that he will share a body to dissect and the cost of buying one was about a guinea. He helped John Hunter with preparations in the morning and took Baillie's anatomical lectures in the afternoon from 2.00 to 4.00 p.m. At 7.00 p.m. he took Mr Hume's lectures on Surgery and Physiology.

5 See the excellent and lively account of John Hunter and his world, Moore, Wendy (2005), *The Knife Man: The Extraordinary Life and Times of John Hunter, Father of Modern Surgery*, New York: Broadway Books.

> My room has two beds in it and in point of situation is not the most pleasant in the world. The Dissecting Room with half a dozen dead bodies in it is immediately above and that in which Mr. Hunter makes preparations is the next adjoining to it, so that you may conceive it to be a little perfumed. There is a dead carcase just at this moment rumbling up the stairs and the Resurrection Men swearing most terribly. I am informed this will be the case most mornings about four o'clock throughout the winter.[6]

John Hunter and his late brother William were amongst the most famous medical men in Enlightenment Europe. Together and separately, over a 40-year period, they were responsible for educating most of the next generation of leading physicians and surgeons in Britain and America. The medical teachings of William and John Hunter affected not just their sensibilities but also those of medical men such as the young James Williams.

William Hunter saw one of his most important roles to be the creator and promoter of a set of dispassionate protocols to deal with his own discomfort – he fainted during operations – and those of his students' with the physical realities of dissecting and surgery. John Hunter, who liaised with bodysnatchers and was himself involved in the practice, expressed a dispassionate attitude towards obtaining, dissecting and treating the human body. Both men helped their students forge professional identities based on a mutual language and the values that they taught and enacted throughout their lives.

We begin with the eldest brother. William Hunter's background was not illustrious; he was born in 1718, the seventh of ten children to a Scottish Presbyterian farmer. Meant for the Church – Hunter miserably attended the Divinity School at the University of Glasgow – he apprenticed himself in 1734 to William Cullen, a local surgeon.[7] Cullen appears to have arranged for Hunter to attend anatomy lectures at the University of Edinburgh. In 1740, armed with introductions from Cullen and others to the leading Scottish practitioners of surgery and man-midwifery in London, Hunter departed for the capital and became first a pupil of William Smellie, and then anatomy assistant to James Douglas.[8] Hunter was also made tutor to Douglas's son, William George. Dr Douglas entered William Hunter as a surgical pupil at St George's Hospital under the direction of James Wilkie. Although James Douglas died in 1742, Hunter continued living in the Douglas home for several years and took over many of Douglas's patients. In 1743 Hunter and William George travelled to Paris where the teaching of anatomy was considered to be more advanced.[9] There they attended a course of about 80 anatomical lectures given by the physician Antoine Ferrein and the surgeon H.F. Le Dran at the Collège Royal from mid-November 1743 to late-March 1744.[10]

---

6 Dobson, Jesse (1969), *John Hunter*, Edinburgh: E. & S. Livingstone Ltd., p. 178.

7 Hunter attended the University from the age of 13 to 18. See Beekman, Fenwick, (1944) 'William Hunter's Education at Glasgow', *Bulletin of the History of Medicine*, 55 (3), pp. 284–97.

8 Smellie, like Hunter, was from Lanarkshire.

9 William George Douglas died at age 30 'from dissolute habits.' Simmons, p. 13.

10 Gelfand, Toby (1988), 'The 'Paris Manner' of Dissection: Student Anatomical Dissection in Early Eighteenth-Century Paris', *Bulletin of the History of Medicine*, 46 (2), pp.

Anatomical instruction was offered in Paris at the Schools of Medicine and Surgery, the Jardin du Roi, the Collège Royal, the major hospitals and privately. The city was renowned as a place where bodies were available for medical teaching and hence was an attractive study destination for budding surgeons.[11] The anonymous author of *A Short Comparative View of the Practice of Surgery in the French Hospitals* (1740) exclaimed:

> It is generally said in *England*, among the Common People, and sometimes among the Learned, That a Man cannot be a good *Surgeon* and *Accoucheur*, without a Tour to *Paris*.[12]

William Hunter appears to have been deeply influenced by the practice of dissection and the teaching of anatomy in France. On his return to London in 1746, he placed an advertisement in several newspapers announcing a course of medical lectures, where the 'Paris manner' of dissection would be used in instruction. Hunter was implying that, contrary to the practice at the Company of Surgeons' Hall where each apprentice simply got to watch a dissection, he would provide the attendees of his lectures with their very own cadavers to dissect.[13] Christopher Lawrence has described Hunter as one of the founders of the literature devoted to 'characterizing any form of anatomy teaching that was not based on the Paris Manner as second rate.'[14]

The spread of anatomy schools, first in Paris and then in London, particularly increased the prestige of surgery. There were at least 27 lecturers in anatomy working in London before William Hunter opened up for business in 1746.[15] However he quickly became the best known of them all. Besides instructing young men in the art and science of medicine Hunter's smooth manners and eloquent speech attracted a diverse audience, including such noted Enlightenment figures as Adam Smith, Edward Gibbon, Edmund Burke, William Robertson and Tobias Smollett. The historian Gibbon would not leave London during the winter of 1777 because he was

---

99–130, see p.103.

11 Ibid., p. 104.

12 Anonymous (1740), *A Short Comparative View of the Practice of Surgery in the French Hospitals,* London, p. 4. The work was attributed to the surgeon John Harrison by an anonymous French author. See the abridged translation in (1843), *Le Moniteur les hôpitaux*, VI, pp. 1241–5 and 1249–52.

13 The Company of Barber-Surgeons separated in 1745. William Chesleden was one of the leaders in the movement to break up the Company and dissociate barbery from surgery.

14 Lawrence, Christopher (1988), 'Alexander Monro *Primus* and the Edinburgh Manner of Anatomy', *Bulletin of Medical History*, 62, pp. 193–214, quotation from p. 194. Johanna Geyer-Kordesch and Fiona MacDonald point out that Hunter's new teaching methods were influenced by Glasgow anatomical teaching in the early 1740s especially given his and William Cullen's close relationship with the Hamilton family. See (1999), *The History of the Royal College of Physicians and Surgeons of Glasgow 1599–1858, Physicians and Surgeons in Glasgow*, London: The Hambledon Press, p. 223. Perhaps advertising anatomy teaching in the 'Paris Manner' had more marketing cachet than in the 'Glasgow Manner'?

15 For details on lecturers in London in the eighteenth century see, Lawrence, Susan (1996), *Charitable Knowledge: Hospital pupils and practitioners in eighteenth-century London*, Cambridge: Cambridge University Press.

attending William Hunter's lectures for two hours daily, 'which have opened to me a new and very entertaining scene *within myself*.'[16]

Until his death in 1783, William Hunter combined a career as an anatomist with that of a fashionable accoucheur or man-midwife. His patients included the Pitts, the Fitzroys, the Earl of Sandwich, Lord North, the Coutts, the Hollands and Queen Charlotte. His friends included Tobias Smollett, Dr Johnson, Henry Fielding, Horace Walpole and David Hume. In 1777 Edward Gibbon and Adam Smith attended his lectures.[17] Glasgow University gave William Hunter an MD in 1750 and he maintained strong ties with the faculty there throughout his life. They sent him both pupils and assistants. In 1756 Hunter was disenfranchised from the Company of Surgeons for the fee of 40 guineas. This allowed him, like Daniel Turner, to apply to become a Licentiate of the College of Physicians. In this Hunter was successful but he was denied the honour of becoming a Fellow. There were two reasons for this decision: his degree was not from Oxbridge and he was a man-midwife and therefore classified as an undesirable manual labourer. Enraged, Hunter joined with other 'foreign' graduates in the capital, and after an abortive attempt to storm a meeting of the College of Physicians they turned to litigation. In 1771 the College caved in and allowed Scottish graduates to apply for fellowship but they still barred accoucheurs or man-midwives like Hunter. But by 1771 William Hunter may have not cared, for by then he was the most famous and wealthiest medical lecturer in Britain.

Among the various types of medical training available in London private anatomy schools set up by individuals were the most popular. Several reasons contributed to their success. First the students only needed cash to attend, and no evidence of prior training or education was required. Second the access to high-grade preparations and anatomical models as teaching aids was a great attraction. Third the lectures embodied new discoveries: 'Hunter's auditors heard of his research on aneurism, the placental circulation, the lymphatic system and the gravid uterus, nowhere available in print.'[18] This commercial approach to learning proved to be so popular that by 1800 at least 40 per cent of all provincial practitioners had obtained some of their medical education in London.[19]

William Hunter's course was easily the most elaborate at 112 two-hour lectures held six days a week from 2.00–4.00 p.m., October to May (summer was avoided due to the rapid decay of the bodies used in lectures). Hunter's school also offered instruction in a multitude of medical subjects other than anatomy. Of the 112

16 Dobson, p. 177. She gives no reference. On the Enlightenment fascination with the body, especially the nerves, see Benfield, Barker, G. (1992), *The Culture of Sensibility: Sex and Society in Eighteenth Century Britain*, Chicago: University of Chicago Press.

17 Moore, p. 43.

18 Porter, Roy (March 1995), 'Medical Lecturing in Georgian London', *The British Journal of the History of Science*, 28 (96), pp. 91–9, quotation from p. 94. Lawrence, *Charitable Knowledge*, sums up: 'As medical men offered their ideas and experiences primarily to their peers, they began the process of claiming autonomy for their medical practice, distinct from the views of patients, irregular competitors, and past-practitioners. Reputations were formed by turning to other medical men for approval rather than socially respectable patients and natural philosophers and natural historians.' p. 27.

19 Porter, 'Medical Lecturing', p. 96.

meetings, 2 were introductory, 80 were on anatomy, 15 on operative surgery, 3 on making preparations and embalming, and the remaining 12 on midwifery.[20] From 1768 the lectures were given in Hunter's purpose-built anatomy theatre in his lavish home in Great Windmill Street. There he trained among others, his brother John, William Hewson, William Cumberland Cruikshank and his nephew Matthew Baillie. Indeed using the terms of a man-midwife, William Hunter prided himself on being 'a breeder of anatomists'.[21]

John Hunter had a long and somewhat difficult association with his brother. In 1748 he came down to London from Scotland and was then employed as William's primary assistant until 1760.[22] During this period John experimented and published research on the relationship of form to function in the human and animal body.[23] He also studied with William Cheselden at the Chelsea Hospital from 1749 to 1750. The following year John became a pupil of the eminent surgeon Percivall Pott at St Bartholomew's. Three years later he entered St George's Hospital as a surgeon's pupil and for five months in 1756 acted as a house surgeon until he resigned, probably to spend more time in his brother's dissecting room.[24]

During the 1750s the brothers collaborated and published findings on the tubules and descent of the testes, the human lachrymal ducts, congenital hernias and the lymphatic system. Their findings on the placenta and maternal circulation led to arguments over who discovered what and when and led to hostility between the two that was never fully resolved. In 1760 John left his brother's employ and became an army surgeon. He saw action during the Seven Years War (1756–63) in Normandy and Portugal, and his conservative approach to treating missile injuries was published posthumously in 1794.

---

20 The students paid approximately seven guineas each for the course and Hunter frequently had over 100 attend. See Lane (2001), *A Social History of Medicine: Health, healing and disease in England, 1750–1950*, London: Routledge, p. 28.

21 William Hunter boasted of having 'bred' John Hunter to practical anatomy and William Hewson, and William Cruikshank to anatomy, in Simmons, *Two Introductory Lectures*, p.60. This phrase occurs elsewhere in his students' lecture notes. Matthew Baillie took William Hunter's course in anatomy and John Hunter's in surgery from 1780–83. He also became a perpetual student at St George's and eventually was appointed both surgeon and physician at the hospital. Baillie was also a lecturer at the Windmill Street school until 1799. Cruikshank had been at the school since 1771 and, with Baillie, took over the school on William Hunter's death in 1783. William and John Hunter were his uncles.

22 Paget, Stephen (1897), *John Hunter: Man of Science and Surgeon*, London: T. Fisher Unwin. Another son, James, had gone to live with William and assist in the dissecting room. He died in 1743 of phthisis at age 29 probably from his work, p. 21.

23 What we would term physiology. His three main treatises were (1771), *Natural History of the Human Teeth On Venereal Disease*, London, (1786), *A Treatise on Venereal Disease*, London and (1794), *A Treatise on the Blood Inflammation and Gun-shot Wounds*, London.

24 Susan Lawrence's *Charitable Knowledge* masterfully surveys hospital medicine in the eighteenth century. She states that 11,059 pupils signed up to walk the wards between 1725 and 1815, p. 108. Governors took over moral and character questions which were once exercised with the apprentices by the Masters, p. 126 (especially after 1745 when apprenticeship was no longer a prerequisite for exam for surgeons).

John Hunter returned to London in 1763 on half pay from the army with no other work. William Hewson was now working in his old job and Hunter turned to supplementing his army pension by working with a dentist, James Spence.[25] He also established a surgical practice from his home. In 1765 Hunter purchased two acres of land at Earls Court where he built a country retreat and a home for his vast menagerie of lions, tigers, buffalo, birds, fish, snakes and insects.[26] He was elected a Fellow of the Royal Society in 1767, became a member of the Company of Surgeons in 1768, and was elected surgeon to St George's Hospital the same year. He finally opened his own anatomy school in Jermyn Street, London in 1770.[27] There he lectured on all maladies, not just those related to surgery. John Hunter had hundreds of students, including Edward Jenner, Astley Cooper, Anthony Carlisle and John Abernethy.[28] John Hunter's American pupils included Philip Syng Physic, William Shippen and John Morgan. Besides courses at his school, Hunter taught a thousand or more students in practical surgery during his lifetime at St George's Hospital. In 1783 he moved his school, museum and dissecting room to two houses and a vacant lot he had bought on Leicester Street and Castle Street.[29] Hunter offered 86 one-hour evening lectures three times a week from October–April. His audience included Joseph Banks, Captain Cook, James Watt and the Astronomer Royal, Dr Nevil Maskelyne.

John Hunter was very different from William. He could be coarse and prided himself on his lack of genteel learning. The eighteenth century was the age of clubbing and John valued meeting in small groups to discuss research and medical news. He helped found two societies in 1783 and 1785. The *Society for the Improvement of Medical and Chirugical Knowledge* published some findings in its *Transactions* and met once a month at Slaughter's Coffee House. The *Lyceum Medicum Londonenses for the Advancement of Medical Knowledge* met monthly at his London home.[30] Hunter's personality is captured in the following exchange between himself and Dr Marshal at one of the meetings of the *Society for Improvement*:

> Having mentioned at a meeting of this Society, that, in the dissection of those who had died insane, he [Marshal] had always found marks of disease in the head. Mr. Hunter

25 His work with Spence is reflected in *Treatise on the Natural History of the Human Teeth*, 1771. See Moore for details.

26 Like William Harvey, John Hunter was given access to the King's deer in Richmond Park. He experimented with tying off their antlers and made discoveries about collateral circulation as a result. See his *Observations on Certain Parts of the Animal Oeconomy*.

27 William Hunter vacated Jermyn Street when he moved to Great Windmill Street and John appears to have taken over his offices there.

28 All became important surgeons at leading London hospitals. Cooper went to Guy's, Abernethy to Barts, Cline to St Thomas' and Carlisle to the Westminster. Morgan and Shippen founded the first medical school in America in Philadelphia.

29 Now Leicester Square and Charing Cross Road.

30 On medical publications in the eighteenth century see Rousseau, G.S. (1999) '"Stung in to action ...": Medicine Professionalism, and the News', in Raymond, Joad (ed.), *News, Newspapers, and Society in Early Modern Britain*, London: Frank Cass and Company, pp. 176–205. On medical societies see Lawrence, *Charitable Knowledge*, p. 20.

> denied the truth of this in very coarse language. The other members interfering, Mr. Hunter agreed to say, that his expressions did not refer to Dr. Marshal's veracity, but to the accuracy of his observations. Marshal, not being satisfied with this declaration, at the next meeting of the Society demanded an ample apology; but Mr. H. instead of making one, repeated the offensive expressions; on which Marshal poured some water over his head out of a bottle which stood near them. A scuffle ensued, which was immediately stopped by other members, and no further personal contention between them ever occurred. But Marshal, conceiving that their common friends in the Society had, from the superior rank of Mr. Hunter, favoured him more in this matter than justice permitted, soon after estranged himself from them.[31]

If we now turn back to William, John's elder brother by ten years, a different picture emerges – of a man concerned with his image as a gentlemanly anatomist and accoucheur, and of a gifted teacher but one who fainted at the sight of blood and rarely practised surgery as a result.

William Hunter and the shaping of boys into medical men

To guard his success from being copied by others William Hunter never published any of his lectures during his lifetime. Upon his death in 1783, however, his executors found a heavily annotated manuscript, *Two Introductory Lectures by Dr. Hunter. Read at his New Theatre on the first and second day of October, 1767*. The lectures, related to the history and uses of anatomy and were subsequently published by his trustees in 1784. From this source and surviving notes taken by students at his lectures it is possible to reconstruct partially how Hunter actually taught the subjects of anatomy, surgery and midwifery. Hunter incorporated much of his own research into the lectures on topics such as the differences between frog and human blood and why it is more difficult to revive animals than humans after drowning.[32] He also discussed something that had interested Pepys – whether a hanged man dies of asphyxia or from blood being cut off from the brain and how much pain ensues in either case.

The several extant versions of the lectures show that Hunter was aware, like Duverney, that a major part of shaping a medical man rested in addressing the emotions of his pupils. Perhaps he remembered hearing advice in Paris about the utility of cutting on the dead to prepare oneself for cutting on the living? Hunter characterized anatomic inquiry as 'the passive submission of dead bodies' and lectured that:

---

31 Wade, Nicholas J. (2005), 'Medical Societies and Insanity in Late-Eighteenth Century London: The Fight between Andrew Marshal and John Hunter', *Journal of the History of the Neurosciences*, 14, pp. 11–15. This is from the obituary of Andrew Marshal (1742–1813) and describes a meeting of the Society for the Improvement of Medical and Chirurgical Knowledge in 1789.

32 See for example, Anonymous (*c.*1770), *Notes of lectures by William Hunter*, Royal College of Surgeons, MS 42.c, ff. 28–9.

> It is dissection alone that can teach us, where we may cut the living body, with freedom & dispatch; and where we may venture, with great circumspection and delicacy, and where we must not, upon any account attempt it. This informs the *head*, gives dexterity to the *hand*, and familiarises the *heart* with a sort of *necessary inhumanity*, the use of cutting instruments upon our fellow-creatures.[33]

This passage appears with slightly different wording in notes taken by Hunter's students:

> Anatomy is the basis of Physic and Surgery, it teaches him where to cut with safety and dispatch and enables him to form a just prognostic of a disease, in short, anatomy is the basis of surgery it informs the head, guides the hand, and familiarises the heart with *a kind of necessary inhumanity* in the use of cutting instruments.[34]

Analyzing Hunter's lectures and his students' responses to them helps reveal what he meant by necessary inhumanity and how this relates to dispassion.

William Hunter seems to have always begun his course of 112 lectures with advice not to miss a single lecture, as it breaks 'the chain of things'. He further explained that:

> Upon this account, I think it injudicious for a beginner to write notes in the time of lecture. His business is first of all to get clear ideas of everything. His eyes and ears are to be employed in that service only. He is first to understand; let him remember as he can.[35]

In fact, Hunter suggested that his students attend a second course of the same lectures if they wished to acquire – as he modestly put it – 'a reference book for life'. Learning how to take notes was important in developing a 'talent of writing for the public ... to protect and justify [one's] conduct in the medical profession.'[36] His preference was for a student who had not read many books at all, 'for he will come with no false, no confused ideas in his head, and therefore will have no rubbish to be cleared away.'[37]

---

33 Simmons, p. 67. Also see Anonymous, *Introductory Lecture of Mr William Hunter*, St. Thomas's Hospital, MS 55, f. 182v. Simmons was a member of the Society of Physicians and read a eulogy at the first meeting after Hunter's death, although he barely knew William Hunter. Helen Brock transcribed the copy of the memoir in Glasgow Library which is in the hand of John Hunter. She surmises that John was unhappy with Simmons's attempt to eulogise his brother. As Brock points out in the introduction, 'Simmons's Life of Dr. William Hunter is still looked upon as an official biography. It was but an evening's talk and necessarily a very brief account. John's additions of much hitherto unknown material adds immeasurably to its value.' Simmons titled his published version, *An Account of the Life and Writings of the late William Hunter*, London, 1783.

34 William Hunter (1775), *Anatomical Lectures*, f. 9r, New York Academy of Medicine, the hand has not been identified. Italics mine.

35 .Simmons, p. 103.

36 Ibid., p. 107.

37 Ibid., p. 108. There is an obvious reference to John Locke's notion of the mind as a blank slate. Similar advice to Hunter's occurs twice in the first 12 pages of Alexander Monro (1763), *Praelectiones on Anatomy & Surgery,* MS. 42.d., ff. 9 & 11. Also see, *Anatomical*

Conscious that plunging into dissecting on the first day of lecture, 'might even create disgust to a study from which [they] ought to receive pleasure and advantage', William Hunter first had his students observe their own bodies. To demonstrate the colour blood gives to the skin, for example, he encouraged them to hold their arms down and watch their hands turn red from the blood draining. Hunter eased his students into dissecting through such demonstrations. He showed some of his intricate handmade preparations in order to rouse their curiousity about what could be found in the body and how it could be preserved. Hunter established strict parameters for how the preparations might be viewed to restrict the impact the preserved parts could have on the students. Not only were they to be passed right to left in the front row and left to right on the second in an orderly fashion, only the area of the preparation Hunter directed them to was to be observed – or they would 'speculate too much on other parts' and develop 'strange fancies'.[38] From the beginning of the course, thus he attempted to consciously rein in their passions and promote a moderate response to the human body. Rules were important in forming a cohesive body of medical men. Hunter drew their explicit attention to the 'conditions ... hung up in a frame' in the dissecting room.[39]

Ironically given all this focus on discipline and the whetting of appetites for becoming a surgeon, William Hunter himself was squeamish of operations. His brother John revealed in 1784 that the most well-known anatomy teacher to that time:

> At first ... practiced both surgery and midwifery, but to the former of these he always had an aversion *because he hated operations, would often faint at an operation, even disliked to bleed, although he studied how the art might be improved.*[40]

What was it Hunter 'hated' about operations? The quotation suggests he had the fairly common phobia of turning faint when seeing blood flow from a body. Knowing this, his words regarding the reason to dissect – to acquire a necessary inhumanity – take on a plaintive tone. As Hunter strove to instil a dispassionate demeanor in his students so they could cut on the living, he was also struggling with his own inability to do so. He certainly appears to have presented himself as cool and calm to the point that it was publicly satirized. At the request of Martin Van Butchell, a former pupil of his who became a well-known and eccentric dentist, Hunter embalmed his wife.[41] She

Lectures delivered by Sir Joseph Else, Surgeon from October 1774–April 1775 at his new anatomical Theatre in St. Thomas Hospital. The notes were written by a student identified only as Gardiner.

38 Ibid., p. 111. For example Hunter showed a human gullet with a half crown stuck in it, Anonymous, *Introductory Lecture*, MS 55, f.400r.

39 Ibid., pp. 111–13.

40 Ibid., p. 7.

41 Ernst Gottfried Baldinger, Professor of Medicine at Marburg University published an account of his role in preserving Mrs Van Butchell in (1788), *Medicinisches Journal*, Göttingen, pp. 3–13. 'On the Proper Modes of examining dead Bodies' recounts that 'under his [Hunter's] Direction and assistance I made the Experiment on a Gentlewoman in this city (Mrs van Butchell): she died of Pulmonary Consumption about 4 o' Clock in the Afternoon,

was kept in a glass case in Van Butchell's drawing room and he charged admission to view her. When the dentist remarried, his new wife, not surprisingly, did not want the first Mrs Van Butchell in residence. Under protest he donated his first wife to the Royal College of Surgeons. Satirical verses written by Sir Richard Jebb were circulated as to what skill William Hunter had actually employed to produce such a lifelike Mrs Van Butchell:

> To do his wife's dead Corps peculiar Honour
> Van Butchell wish'd to have it turned to stone,
> Hunter just cast his Gorgon looks upon her,
> And in a twinkling see the thing is done.[42]

Regarding the need to acquire dispassion, Hunter recommended Lorenz Heister's *A General System of Surgery* (1745). Heister was Professor of Physic and Surgery at the University of Helmstadt and a Fellow of the Royal Society and the Royal Academy of Paris. His large folio on surgery was probably the most popular book on surgery in mid-eighteenth-century Britain.[43] Heister was blunt about the traumatic effects of performing surgery and the need to acquire clinical dispassion:

> The Students in Surgery should not only be furnished with Strength of Body, but Constancy of Mind also, that they may remain unmolested and unmoved by the Stench, Blood, Pus, and Nastiness that will naturally occur to them in their Practice; they should consider that

---

et we went there by 6 o' Cl. on the same Evening.' Turpentine and vermillion were injected into the arteries and 'There was a beautiful blush over the whole Body ... . It was washed all over with the essential Oil, and put on a Bed of 140 of Paris Plaister (which was a View to the absorption of moisture) in a mahogany oblong Box. For the first 7 Month the Body looked os (sic) if it were asleep and a little warm from the Blush upon it; but it has since gradually lost this appearance, and gets every Day more and more of the Look of a Mummy. The Vessels, particularly of the Tibia, still look most beautiful as if in ice.' pp. 9–11. In 1779 Hunter embalmed the daughter of the Spanish Ambassador. I thank Katherine Bell for sending me Baldinger's account from Budapest.

42 Simmons, p. 55. Unfortunately, Mrs Van Butchell was one of the many Hunterian preparations destroyed in the bombing of the Royal College of Surgeons in London during the Second World War. Martin Van Butchell studied under both Hunters and was a dentist, truss and garter maker. He made false teeth for William Hunter out of ivory walrus tusk in 1772 and again in 1776. He was an eccentric figure. 'The senior Van Butchell became tremendously upset in his latter days by the fact that the men in England were not permitting their beards to grow. To this practice he allotted the pusillanimity of the race, citing the story of Samson and Delilah for confirmation. It was his habit to ride about on Sundays, wearing heavy dark rimmed spectacles with his beard trailing toward the ground, on a white pony which he not infrequently decorated with large splotches of purple paint. His son was the first surgeon to be sued in England on the death of a patient for malpractice.' Beekman, Fenwick , *Hunteriana*, Vol. III in the New York Academy of Medicine. Also, Haslam, Fiona (1996), *From Hogarth to Rowlandson: Medicine in Art in Eighteenth-Century Britain*, Liverpool: Liverpool University Press, pp. 240–47.

43 Not all praised Heister. For example, see negative comments by Charles Nicholas Jenty in his three-volume work (1757), *A Course of Anatomico-Physiological Lectures on the Human Structure and Animal Oeconomy*, London, *passim.*

by frequent exercise these things will become customary to them, and they will acquire another nature as it were.[44]

Smelling disease and decay came first in Heister's list of what could unsteady the hand, heart and mind of a medical man just as it had for Harvey. Heister's point that surgery was no place for the weak and fanciful was hammered home in a series of examples:

Dr. WALTER HARRIS, in his eighth chirurgical Dissertation, openly condemns this Operation, [removing an aneurism] and calls it dreadful and rash Butchery; but for what reasons himself best knows. He seems, in my Opinion, to have been a very timorous Physician, who, out of Fear, or a foolish and ill-grounded Compassion, is for rejecting some of the most considerable and useful Operations in Surgery.[45]

Heister's statement that one would naturally develop 'another nature as it were' through surgery was not exactly the same as Hunter's method of familiarizing his students' hearts to 'a sort of necessary inhumanity'. The former required only repeated experience of dissecting, but the latter required an active teaching program.

To counteract the timidity and fearfulness of the young medical student, Hunter devised his program of 112 lectures to stress constantly the necessity to hone acute observation and manual dexterity through repetitive dissection. Surgery required discipline and a physical familiarity with the material aspects of medicine – instruments, skeletons and organs. As a fellow London accoucheur, William Rowley, aptly phrased it, 'Dissection leaves an impression in the mind never to be effaced.'[46] He also echoed the gloomy words of Thomas Bartholin quoted in Chapter One on the misery of learning anatomy and the heroic effort it took to persist in handling corpses. Rowley characterized those who fell in this task as martyrs:[47]

Cannot get knowledge of anatomy from books / specimens / engravings No: the student who would wish to discharge his duties with a conscientious rectitude, must repeatedly with his own hands, dissect dead human bodies; must breathe for many

44 Heister, Lorenz (1745), *A General System of Surgery*, London, p. 24.

45 Simmons, p. 303.

46 Rowley, William (1795), *On the Absolute Necessity of Encouraging, Instead of Preventing or Embarrassing the Study of Anatomy. With a Plan to Prevent Violating the Dormitories of the Defunct. Addressed to the Legislature of Great Britain*, London, footnote, p. 17. Rowley was Physician to the 'St. Mary-Le-Bone Infirmary'. He attacked Hunter in (1774), *A Letter to Dr. William Hunter ... on the Dangerous Tendency of Medical Vanity, occasioned by the death of the late Lady Holland*, London. Hunter had treated Lady Holland in 1768 for a painful uterine discharge. Rowley accused him of being too proud and inhumane to call him in when the cure failed. It seems Hunter had advised the friends of Lady Holland not to call Rowley in as it might increase her pain. This, Rowley claimed, had affected his reputation and Hunter must publicly apologize. On Hunter's attitude to other medical men see Simmons. 'In consultation with his medical brethren, he delivered his opinions with diffidence and candour', p. 67 and 'No man was ever more tenacious than Dr. Hunter of what he conceived to be his anatomical rights', p. 24.

47 The perceived and unperceived dangers of the dissecting room are discussed further in Chapter Six.

> months in the unpleasant, and frequently destructive air of a dissecting room; he must risk his own life to be serviceable to others; and frequently some of the brightest ornaments of the profession have fallen victims to their ardour in these necessary though horridly disagreeable pursuits.[48]

Hunter regarded knowledge of physiology and pathology as particularly important because this guaranteed diagnostic accuracy and enhanced the ability to devise new surgical techniques. Pictures told lies unless they were truly drawn from nature. Looking at a drawing of the anatomy of the body was not enough to ensure knowledge, and therefore confidence, in operating; neither was merely describing the structure of the parts. Instead the student must have it demonstrated to him. Hunter criticized an illustration from his favoured surgical text by comparing it to the opened body laying in front of the audience:

> I must here shew a fault in the plate of Heister that has been so much confided in that Le Dran in a work of his own just copied it over– This shews the rectum at a considerable distance from the under side of the prostrate and bladder, so that guided by this plate we will think there is sufficient room for the knife to cut through the prostrate without going near the gut– This may have bad consequences for you see in nature they lie close together– so I would always have you guided by nature.[49]

Hunter had seen Le Dran dissect and vivisect in Paris. For Hunter, nature gave 'solid knowledge, arising from the information of his own senses. Hence his ideas are clear and make a lasting impression upon his memory.'[50] Repeatedly seeing (getting the theory) and manipulating (getting the practice) multiple insensible bodies was the only way to gain a free and familiar hand. Over and over again, Hunter used the word 'freedom' in his lectures. It seems to have represented both the freedom from sensibility of a corpse and the freedom this then gave to the students to probe and thrust with their hands or instruments in the body. Conceptually both meanings can be seen in the following passage on catheter insertion:

> Introducing the catheter [into the penis] is difficult in an unexperienced hand, but easy in an experienced hand, after understanding its theory, to become expert at it we should practice frequently on the dead and then on living Bodies.[51]

Pain, of course, precluded a medical man from moving freely about the living body. William Hunter addressed the issue of pain in two ways in his anatomy lectures to students. First, he put forward the traditional argument that surgeons ill-trained in anatomy are little more than butchers:

48 Rowley, p. 6.

49 Anonymous, *Notes taken from Dr. William Hunter's Lectures c.*1783, College of Physicians, Philadelphia, MS 10a/63, f. 201r. Caspar Witstar may have bought these notes while in England in 1784. Wistar became a physician in Philadelphia and President of the American Philosophical Society. He published a *System of anatomy for the use of students of medicine*, 1811–14.

50 Simmons, p. 87.

51 Anonymous, *Notes taken from*, f. 202v.

> In the hands of a good Anatomist, surgery is a salutary, a divine art; but when practiced by men who know not the structure of the human body, it often becomes barbarous and criminal.[52]

This is one of the few places where Hunter mentions any religious purpose to dissecting.[53] More typically, he framed his remarks in the second way, within strictly anatomical terms. Lecturing on the nature of pain led Hunter to muse on our delusion that somehow we think we understand what is, after all, only a purely physiological process:

> When any part is hurt, we can say very exactly where the painful sensation is. Think this is entirely by habit – There is nothing in the nature of pain or the sensation itself that could tell us where it is, thus when a pain is run into any part of the surface of our body we who are grown up can from the pain tell exactly where it is – But this is from experience alone, for an infant when any part is hurt feels pain but knows not from what part the sensation comes, till it learns to judge by experience.[54]

Hunter then used the famous Cartesian example of the child who keeps putting his hand into the candle flame until he works out the connection between his hand, the burning sensation and the flame. He concluded that:

> But as the internal parts are not objects of seeing and handling, our ideas of the seat of pain coming from them is much less distinct than from parts on the surface.[55]

Bodies could not be read by their owners but only by those with training in how to 'see and handle' the interior of the body. For Hunter this meant a precise and painstaking process of cutting, experimenting and vivisecting, made no doubt doubly difficult for him because of his faintness at the sight of blood. Such a theory also denied taking a patient history at face value. Hunter offered many examples to his students of the genre of patients 'who thought they had this but really had that':

> A gentleman had stomach complaints for many Years which he took to be gouty – so he went every year to Bath and drank the water, but at length they failed and the complaint increased – I saw him at this time, and among other complaints he told me his stools were black ... this made me suspect they were not real faeces but blood – I poured water on them and shook them in it, and they gave it a bloody tinge – hence I thought there was a bleeding vessel within him.[56]

Hunter had established the truth of his diagnosis. Unfortunately, the patient's physician was, 'fond of the strabiliarian doctrine and said this was black bile, and prescribed purges to carry it off.'[57] As Daniel Turner pitted his surgical knowledge

52 Ibid., f. 68r.

53 William was a Whig and a Deist, John a Tory and a Presbyterian. William appears to have become more of a Tory when he was appointed the Royal Accoucheur.

54 Anonymous, *Notes taken from*, f. 427v.

55 Ibid., f. 428r.

56 Ibid., f. 412r.

57 *Idem.*

against a ‘Chymist’, Hunter pitted his new experimental diagnosis against the old theoretical doctrine of the patient’s physician. Hunter proclaimed that he did not support the ancients’ notion of the existence of black (or yellow) bile because ‘we know no such thing in the body as black bile.’[58] The physician with his belief in the humours won but the patient did not. Hunter stressed to his students what the awful consequences were of ignoring experimental knowledge. He invoked the patient’s corpse as witness:

> ... from my notion of a bleeding vessel I begged [the physician] that the purges at first should be very gentle – he died – and on inspection we found an ulcer in beginning of duodenum immediately on outside of valve of pylorus ... Now whenever we see these black stools we should be very cautious in giving purges or any thing which irritates the Intestines.[59]

Like Daniel Turner, Hunter used case histories as parables for the edification of his students. One of them wrote:

> Among other methods of explaining and illustrating his doctrines, he used frequently to introduce some opposite story or case that had occurred to him in his practice, and few men had acquired a more interesting fund of anecdotes of this kind, or related them in a more agreeable manner. He had a talent of infusing much of his ardour into his pupils.[60]

In another case the truth was that ‘coagulation of blood in the orifices of blood vessels helps to Stop an haemorrhage.’ Hunter illustrated this through an attack on female midwives who he had seen tear away the placenta with their hands and even, ‘scoop away all the coagulated blood formed in the mouth of each vessel’ ... ‘which soon fall to bleeding again’.[61]

Students appreciated William Hunter’s lecture style; William Hamilton wrote to his father Thomas on 22 December 1777, ‘The Dr is an exceedingly good lecturer and vastly plain, he tells me a story with good humour, one or two which he introduced into his lecturers [sic] on Saturday.’[62] Hunter sought to engrave a three-dimensional map of the body in his students’ minds by familiarizing them with every inch of human anatomy. Such was Hunter’s skill in this area that he found it possible even to teach a method of knowing the body by touch alone:

> As this (female) urethra is streight and very short, a catheter is very easily passed thro’ it – to find the orifice is easy yet as it is very disagreeable to women to have these parts uncovered we commonly do it in the dark. The way is to get the point of your finger between the two labia into the vulva then feel for the lower edge of the os pubis just under the symphysis in the angle you will feel the caruncle and the orifice is so wide and

58 Anonymous, *Notes taken from*, f. 379r.

59 Ibid., f. 413r.

60 Simmons, p. 68.

61 Anonymous, *Notes taken from*, f. 413r.

62 Geyer-Kordesch, p. 224. Thomas Hamilton was a friend of William Hunter’s. He was also Professor of Anatomy at Glasgow University.

dilateable that it instantly flies open to the point of a small finger [and then the catheter can be inserted].[63]

Here he provided a powerful image of the uncooperative nature of the patient versus the cooperative nature of her anatomy. With Hunter's map to the structure of the perineum, the urethral tract instantly 'flies open' at the penetration of the trained and dextrous hand.

What was Hunter's attitude toward the female body – dead or alive? Unlike John, William Hunter never married and we have no clear evidence of him being involved in romantic relationships with women.[64] He seems to have seen the matrimonial life as an impediment to anatomizing. William Hewson, his anatomical assistant, wrote to a friend about his marriage and his master's response to it:

> My friend Dr. Hunter was much afraid it would spoil me as an anatomist ... to tell you a secret I do think the doctor's fears are not groundless. I find the living much more agreeable than the dead. My friend the Dr. indeed when he speaks of women, for himself, says to a man of 50 there is no difference.[65]

William was similarly not thrilled about his brother's marriage; at least that is what is implied in the letter John sent to him announcing the happy event:

> Dear Brother, – To-morrow morning at eight o'clock and at St. James's Church, I enter into the Holy State of Matrimony. As that is a ceremony which you are not particularly fond of, I will not make a point of having your company there. I propose going out of Town for a few days; when I come to Town I shall call upon you. Married or not married, ever yours, John Hunter. Jermyn Street, Saturday Evening.[66]

Ludmilla Jordanova has remarked on the notable contrast between the depictions of the mother (dissected and mutilated) and the foetus (tenderly shown) in Hunter's large and beautiful *The Anatomy of the Human Gravid Uterus* (1774).[67] Thirteen

63 Anonymous, *Notes taken from*, f. 342r.

64 He may have been engaged to James Douglas's daughter, Martha Jane, who died while he was in Paris with her brother.

65 Simmons, p. 56. Letter from Hewson to Mr. Powell, 21 August 1770. Hewson married Mary Stevenson, the daughter of Benjamin Franklin's landlady. Two years later Hewson and Hunter fell out and he replaced him with William Cumberland Cruickshank. Hewson opened his own school at 36 Craven Street near Trafalgar Square (where Franklin lodged) and the remains of ten bodies have been found under the basement kitchens). Hewson cut himself during a dissection and died from the ensuing infection in 1774 at the age of 34.

66 Peachey, George (1924), *A Memoir of William and John Hunter*, Plymouth, p. 154. John married a Scottish surgeon's daughter, Anne Home. He had served with her father in the Seven Year's War. They had four children, two of whom died in infancy. Anne was an accomplished poet, and the composer Haydn set several of her texts. See Adams, Aileen K. (1995), 'I am happy in a Wife: A Study of Mrs John Hunter (1714–1801)', Royal College of Surgeons, pp.32–7.

67 Jordanova, Ludmilla (1985), 'Gender, generation and science: William Hunter's obstetrical atlas', in Bynum, William and Porter, Roy (eds), *William Hunter and the Eighteenth Century Medical World* Cambridge and New York: Cambridge University Press, pp. 387–412,

different subjects at various stages in pregnancy were used to represent one normative pregnant woman:

> On the 11th of February – says he – I was so fortunate as to meet with a Gravid Uterus, to which, from that time all the hours have been dedicated which have been at my own disposal. I have been busy in injecting, dissecting, preserving, and shewing it, and in planning and superintending drawings and plaister casts of it.[68]

As the atlas progresses the foetus grows to term while the woman is slowly dismembered. In the final drawing she is shown empty with her dissected womb laying next to her.[69]

What Hunter strove to do with his atlas and in teaching his students was to portray the body accurately and dispassionately, allowing nature to act as the guide. Similar sentiments are found in the six public lectures he gave to the Royal Academy of Arts as the Professor of Anatomy. They survive in a series of rough notes and drafts, written on the backs of envelopes and old letters. Martin Kemp has reconstructed the lectures and notes:

> The perfect work of art in Hunter's opinion must be minutely accurate according to the forms and functions of Nature; only then would it be capable of producing a total empathy in the spectator as compelling as the response stimulated by Nature herself.[70]

Just as in his introductory lectures to anatomy, Hunter pointed out to the audience at the Royal Academy that the workings of the vascular system could be seen in their own bodies. He discussed the relation of the passions to skin colour – warmth, shame and some other passions cause 'the carnation, the red colour', 'fear, fainting and death produce the paleness'.[71] Hunter then showed them the skeleton and had them handle and draw the bones, much as he had his new medical students see and then touch preparations.[72] His enthusiasm for anatomy, its difficulties and its utility was caught in, 'The human body is so wonderfully complex that a mans whole life might usefully be employed in the Study of it.'[73]

As Adrian Wilson comments, 'the man who entered the womb and resolved the anatomy of the placenta was the same man who had most successfully entered the

p.390. The final drawings also resemble Smellie's wood and sawdust manikins. Hunter had studied with Smellie.

68 Simmons, p. 46. Letter from Hunter to Monro Primus in 1751.

69 McGrath, Roberta (2002), *Seeing Her Sex: Medical Archives and the Female Body*, Manchester: Manchester University Press, pp. 63–9. 'No image has more power over the subject than the image of the body; and for the male, perhaps, this is especially true of the female body, the place where his life began. This can be fascinating and threatening.' p. 87.

70 Kemp, Martin (1975), *Dr William Hunter at the Royal Academy of Arts*, Glasgow: University of Glasgow Press, p. 19.

71 The Text of William Hunter's Lectures to the Royal Academy of Arts, 1769–1772, Kemp (ed.), in *Dr. William Hunter*, p. 35.

72 Kemp, pp. 35–7.

73 Ibid., p. 34.

lying-in chamber.'[74] Indeed, Hunter spent much time in his lectures trying to teach his students the proper conduct to gain access to the chamber:

> A proper degree of seeming tenderness and sympathy can never do a man any disservice but often the contrary ... It is not the mere safe delivery of the woman will recommend an accoucheur, but a sagacious, well-conducted behaviour of tenderness, assiduity, and delicacy.[75]

From 1760, such was his success as an accoucheur that Hunter kept his practice limited to the aristocracy and upper-merchant classes by charging new patients the huge fee of ten guineas. He was famously anti-interventionist in that he rarely used forceps or the crochet hook in deliveries. Both Wilson and Jordanova suggest this was, at least, partly due to his clientele, arguing that as man-midwives became more and more involved in normal, as opposed to late and abnormal, deliveries, Hunter and other accoucheurs wished to distance themselves from an earlier generation of instrument-happy surgeons.[76] But it also reflects his skill in knowing the structure of the female body. Echoing centuries of advice that women had slippery bodies and equally slippery minds:

> Authors tell us of odd substances found in the bladder, or passed from it with the urine, as bundles of hair currants – I (once?) saw a stone extracted from a woman that had a bundle of hair for its nucleus – wth. regard to all these appearances the truth is the female urethra is so large & dilateable as easily to admit musket bullets & bundles of hair to pass thro' it into the bladder, and there are women always foolish enough to play such tricks, & all such stories are to be accounted for in this way. Hydatides may be formed in the urinary passages (as in every other part) & passing among the urine, may be mistaken for currants, but if real currant(s), are passed from the bladder they must have first been introduced into it thro' meatus urinarius – you may examine these marvellous stories as nicely as you please, but be always on your guard, for they almost all turn out to be a deception – women especially however candid they may seem, & however little advantage they appear to reap, have in truth an inclination to constantly to play such tricks.[77]

William Cruikshank, first Hunter's pupil, and then a lecturer at his school from 1771, was blunter and cruder in his assessment of female minds and bodies:

74 Wilson, Adrian (1995), *The Making of Man-midwifery: Childbirth in England, 1660–1770*, Cambridge, MA: Harvard University Press, p. 175.

75 Ibid., p. 176.

76 See Wilson and Jordanova.

77 Anonymous, *Notes taken from*, f. 334v. See Laurent Joubert, Ambrose Paré and, of course, William Harvey.

> Menses – on their appearance every Girl thinks herself fit to –.
> The Clitoris Haller says women promise everything when once you can get to tickle their Glans clitoris.
> Furor Uterinus where the unimpregnated uterus is 3 times enlarged more than it ought to be – they want fucking every minute – have no shame left –.[78]

Rather than diagnose pregnancy with a digital examination of the rectum, Hunter cautioned his students that this was an improper practice when treating a lady. Instead they should offer 'some ambiguous answer', prescribe 'some inoffensive medicine' and so 'amuse her a month longer.'[79] Diagnosing pregnancy was difficult in the early stages and in a passage reminiscent of Daniel Turner's anatomical trickery, Hunter advised his students on how to get a glimpse of female anatomy to help confirm it:

> When we suspect a young woman of pregnancy we should in examining her complaints artfully, bring in whether her breasts be fallen flat or not, and so if possible get a sight of them.[80]

Getting the 'sight of something' was everything to Hunter. However he broadened the definition of sight to include touch and manipulation of the body. He taught his students that control and command in medical settings came from polite and firm conduct, being able to visualize spacial relationships in the body and a theoretical knowledge of ailments. William Stark attended Hunter's lectures, and on 8 October 1765 wrote a letter thanking William Hamilton at Glasgow University for encouraging him to take the course:

> I have seen a considerable variety of diseases, I have learnt to interrogate patients with more propriety, and to remember and class their complaints much better than I could do before.[81]

---

78 Anonymous, *Introductory Lect. Mr Cruikshank 2nd Course Saturday Jan.y 20th 1798*, Royal College of Surgeons, MS 131, ff. 220v, 238r and 240v. Cruickshank became a partner in the school in 1783 along with Matthew Baillie on William Hunter's death. He studied the lymphatic system in animals and humans and published *The Anatomy of the Absorbing Vessels of the Human Body* in 1786. The *Dictionary of National Biography* (2000) states he had a considerable practice as a surgeon but his rather nervous temperament stopped him from becoming a successful operator. 'Cruikshank attended Dr. Johnson in his last illness, and was termed by him, in allusion to his benevolent disposition, "a sweet-blooded man".' When Cruikshank was lancing the dying man's legs to reduce his dropsy, Johnson called out to him. 'I want life, and you are afraid of giving me pain – deeper, deeper.' p. 533. Cruikshank's lecture style does not quite match up to this anecdote.

79 Anonymous, *Notes taken from*, f. 472r

80 Ibid., f. 471v. The problem medical men faced in accurately diagnosing pregnancy is also addressed in (*c*.1770), *London Medical Student Notebook*, Wellcome MS 6922. 'Therefore in those early months, when consulted we shd endeavour to satisfy them by some ambiguous answer, order some little things or other to Amuse them a month or two longer; when if required we may be able safely by Examination to determine', f. 72. This advice is repeated on f. 75. From other passages there is evidence that the notes may well have been taken at one of the Hunters' lectures.

81 Geyer-Kordesch, p. 237.

William Hunter shaped the professional identity of hundreds of students. They in turn shaped their students.

In 1777 William M. Williams attended a series of lectures given by William Shippen (1736–1808), who had been newly appointed Professor of Anatomy to the College of Physicians of Philadelphia. He recorded that Dr Shippen began his introductory lecture with a history of anatomy where the avidity of certain individuals were praised:

> Herophilus alone is said to have dissected 700 Bodies. He likewise opened living Bodies of Criminals which tho it was a cruel practice, yet it was not altogether to be discommended for it shews how anxious he was after new discoveries ... .[82]

Hunter had commented favourably on Vesalius, for being uncommonly studious 'often stealing limbs from the Gallows'.[83] Shippen then drew attention to all the discoveries that had been made and are yet to be made. Like William Hunter who proclaimed his passion for anatomy and spoke of it being 'to this day, and must be to the end of time, new, entertaining, useful, and inexhaustible',[84] Shippen found it strange that more did not practise the art, 'it seems strange that Anatomy should be confined to a single Profession, especially as it is a Study that bids fair to bring the greatest Advantages to Mankind.' Why was this the case Shippen mused, 'Want of Subjects, & the Aversion Men have to dissecting Bodies, seem to have been the most probable Causes.' He ended with the telling words that 'few can at first bear to look at them with any degree of composure.'[85]

Shippen then paraphrased William Hunter:

> ... by frequently dissecting dead Bodies, we inform the Head, give dexterity to the Hand, & insure the success of operations on living Bodies. Besides these dissections inform us where we can cut with safety in the living Body, & they instill into us a sort of inhumanity necessary for a proper use of the knife upon our Felllow Creatures. Surgery, in the Hands of a Skilful Anatomist, is a usefull, salutary and divine Art, but practised by the Ignorant, is barbarity & even Criminal.[86]

He advised his students to take nothing on supposition but to 'see everything' and to dissect at every opportunity. 'Dr. Hunter says, "Students should never read till they have seen some Dissections", by this means wrong Notions are prevented.'[87] Shippen quoted Dr Hunter's cases to illustrate his lectures especially when discussing 'Female organs of generation':

---

82 Williams,William M., *Anatomical Lectures taken from Doct. Wm. Shippen Professor of Anatomy in the College of the City of Philadelphia, 1777*. College of Physicians of Philadelphia, MS 10b 89, f. 2v. On Shippen see, Corner, Betsy Copping (1951), *William Shippen, JR.: Pioneer in American Medical Education*, Philadelphia: American Philosophical Society.

83 Anonymous (1775), *Anatomical Lectures*, f. 6r.

84 Simmons, p. 62.

85 Williams, f. 7v.

86 Ibid., f. 9v.

87 Ibid., f. 16r. This advice is repeated on f. 18r.

> A case after a miscarriage where the Lady was feverish & after some days there appeared a General Mortification of the Pudenda in spite of all that was done, the Patient sunk and the parts sloughed away from the lower part of the belly to the back behind, after this mortification stopped she grew better and at last quite recovered: the Dr. (Hunter) shews this whole Vagina in Spirits.[88]

Shippen identified with William Hunter. The public in Philadelphia also appear to have identified him with one of the activites the Hunters were involved in – resurrecting the dead for anatomy teaching purposes. In January 1770 Shippen had a letter published in the *Pennsylvania Chronicle* stating that he was not, as rumoured, a bodysnatcher.

Anatomy teachers such as William Hunter required literally hundreds of corpses a year to keep their schools running profitably. Can we even know how many dead bodies Hunter required? In 1747 he had 15 students at most, but by 1756 he had more than a hundred and began offering the course twice a year. A conservative estimate is that between 1756 and 1783 William Hunter trained perhaps 5,000 students. Of course not all paid the ten guineas to take the longer course in dissection and obtain the privilege of injecting their own corpses. Instead some would have taken the shorter course in dissection that cost one guinea if two students were willing to share the same cadaver, or two guineas if a student wished to have one to himself.[89] In a letter to his father on 1 January 1778, William Hamilton wrote about the problems decaying and scarce bodies caused Hunter and his pupils:

> The Dr is particularly hurried this week as he is afraid his body won't keep, he is on surgery just now, he explained lithotomy and passing [the] catheter today. Bodies are vastly scarce at present, some of the men have been taken up and tried, but I hope this will soon be over … am close employed in the dissecting room. I have got a leg and thigh from the body the Dr showed the operations upon and I had it injected, I should have done it myself but Mr Home said, as it was rather putrid, it was not proper for a first attempt as I should be apt to burst the vessels, and he did it and very well injected it is. I have been employed upon it since Sunday and I have not got to the knee yet. Bodies are vastly scarce, two resurrection men are taken up and all the burying ground is watched so that I am afraid we shall have little dissecting for some time. There is nothing but an arm and my leg in the dissecting room at present.[90]

After the first season of lectures, William Hamilton was put in charge of the dissecting room. From 1779 to 1780 he recorded dissections of 67 persons in the winter: 22 males, 19 females, 11 male and 15 female children. In addition, 23 adults

---

88 Ibid., f. 170v.

89 Keele, Kenneth D. (1965), *William Harvey: The man, the physician, and the scientist*, London and Edinburgh: Thomas Nelson Printers Ltd, p. 330. Also see Lawrence, *Charitable Knowledge*. Shippen's diary shows that in the year he was a resident pupil at Willliam Hunter's anatomy school in Covent Garden (1759), he generally spent eight hours a day dissecting or making preparations, and the evenings operating, or attending William Hunter's lectures. He also 'chatted' with John Hunter who lodged at the school on anatomical matters. Corner, pp. 20–32.

90 Geyer-Kordesch, p. 226.

were dissected to learn the muscles, 8 for operations, 2 to understand the circulatory system, 3 for making preparations. 7 bodies were used for the lecture course that winter.[91]

This chapter began with a letter from the 16-year-old James Williams to his sister Mary in which he described the living conditions at John Hunter's anatomy school. He obviously struggled with the feelings caused by smelling, seeing, cutting up, and sleeping below freshly dug up and decaying corpses. However, he ended his letter with the brave words that, 'There is something horrible in it at first but I am now reconciled.' Williams had heard the bodies being dragged and heaved up the stairs and had no doubt heard and seen the importance of having an ample supply of fresh material for the use of students:

> The dead body cannot be too fresh for dissection; every hour that it is kept, it is losing something of its fitness for anatomical demonstrations; the blood is transnuding, and bringing all the parts nearer to one colour, which takes off the natural and distinct appearence; and putrefaction is advancing, which makes all the fleshy parts tender and indistinct. For these reasons we may conclude, that, except there be an avowed establishment, for a plentiful supply of dead bodies, a truly useful, and complete course of Anatomy, can only be given in a great city.[92]

Hunter bemoaned living in a country where 'liberty disposed the people to licentiousness and outrage, and Anatomists are not legally supplied with dead bodies ... [Due to this situation, he told his pupils that] particular care should be given to avoid giving offence to the populace.'[93] They must be on guard and speak with caution of 'what may be passing in the School, especially with respect to dead bodies'.[94] The next chapter discusses the relationship between secrecy and values, and how boys like James Williams were taught to reconcile the two.

---

91 *Idem*. Duncan enrolled for classes at the Great Windmill St School and enjoyed Dr Baillie's 'very excellent demonstrations'. 4 January 1795, 'my objects in coming to London are pretty well attained, while the frost continues dissection is at an end, and there is nothing else I can study here.' from letter to his father, Andrew Duncan, chair of the Institutes of Medicine in Edinburgh University from 1790–1821.

92 *Two Introductory Lectures delivered by William Hunter ... As they were left corrected for the Press by himself*, London, 1784, p.87.

93 Ibid., p. 113.

94 Ibid., p. 114.

Chapter Six

Conversant with the Dead

> Q. You have been long in the habit of dissecting human subjects. I presume you have dissected more than any man in Europe?—A. I have dissected some thousands during these thirty-three years.[1]

> I only wish Jack *Hunter* Tearguts had had the cutting of Plutarch he understands anatomy better than any of the Ancients hell plunge his knife up to the hilt in a single drive and thrust his fist in. and all in the space of a Quarter of an hour. he does not mind their crying – tho they cry ever so he'll Swear at them & keep then down with his fist & tell that that hell scrape their bones it they don't lay still & be quiet – What the devil should the people in the hospital that have it done for nothing, make such a piece of work for ...[2]

> Jesse Foot accuses me of not understanding the dead languages; but I could teach him that on the dead body which he never knew in any language, dead or living.[3]

> Letter II to Doctor Baillie, August 20, 1796.
> Perhaps I am bolder from having seen less than yourself, or, as I would willingly suppose from having examined carcinomatous tumours immediately after their removal in the living subject, while you have been principally conversant with the dead.[4]

In 1724 the physician William Stukeley gave an eyewitness account of a debate in the House of Lords. It was over the passage of a bill to allow the College of Physicians

---

1 John Hunter testifying as an expert witness for the defence at the *Trial of John Donellan, Esq., for the wilful Murder, by poison of Sir Theodosius Edward Allesley Boughton, Bart., at the Assizes at Warwick, on Friday, March 20, 1781.* His evidence that Sir Allesley had died of a stroke and not from being poisoned with laurel water did not help get John Donellan off. He was sentenced to hanging three days later.

2 Blake lived around the corner from John Hunter from 1782–84 at 23 Green St. William Blake (1987), *An Island in the Moon, A Facsimile of the Manuscript Introduced, Transcribed and Annotated by Michael Phillips*, Cambridge and New York: Cambridge University Press, pp. 39–40.

3 Paget, Stephen (1897), *John Hunter: Man of Science and Surgeon*, London: T. Fisher Unwin, p. 234, quoting John Hunter on Jesse Foot.

4 Adams, Joseph (1801), *Observations on the Cancerous Breast*, London, p. 28. Adams was a physician on the island of Madeira. He corresponded with Baillie, Cline, Babington, Abernethy and Stokes. Like all of them he had attended William and John Hunters' lectures. Adams was interested in the nature of cancer and believed it was alive like John Hunter had claimed hydatids were. He wrote to all of his colleagues asking for permission to obtain and publish letters regarding cases they have seen to support his thesis and also obtain drawings of amputated breasts for publication. Letter II to Doctor Baillie, August 20, 1796.

to collect more executed bodies from Tyburn Fields, the public hanging grounds outside London. The College was also hoping to have its powers strengthened to resist the family and friends who often fought with them at Tyburn when they tried to take the bodies. The various reactions of the ruling class to the bill was instructive, ranging from disgust at the topic, to ironic support for the 'mobb' trying to seize the corpses, to concern that the body of a Lord might be turned over to the physicians rather than decently buried, to a deafening silence from the ecclesiastics:

> Ld. Townsend said, in relation to the Anatomy clause, that the mobb show'd a merciful disposition in hindring dissections, and it ought to be encourag'd. [Townsend was Viscount Charles 1676–1738, the chief minister before Robert Walpole] Ld. Carteret wondr'd how that clause was foisted into the bill, that it was a subject not to be nam'd in the house of Lords. Ld. Trevor sd. it was taking away a prerogative of the Crown, for it might be the misfortune of a person of consideration to be convicted of capital crimes, & then the King could not dispose of his body, upon which they all rejected it. The Bps. [Bishops] said not one word all the time.[5]

Stukeley was very disappointed with the debate, largely because nobody had recognized the importance and nobility of dissection in medical education. He ends his account by commenting on the relation of anatomy to medical power:

> I found there was a general indifference as to the bill in the whole house, & as to Anatomy all the fine things that might have been said by anyone in its favours, were entirely dropp'd. The Lds. it seems were unwilling to trust any one with power, & that the Physicians, (they imagin'd,) had some sinister end in it.[6]

This concern had disappeared by the passing of the Murder Act of 1752. It specifically laid down that dissection was now part of the punishment, and anyone seeking to rescue a body from the surgeons at the gallows was subjected to deportation. Dissection was prescribed as a 'further Terror and peculiar mark of Infamy' for the 'better preventing the horrid Crime of Murder' that was thought to be on a meteoric

---

5 Surtees Society (1882), *The Family Memoirs of the Rev. William Stukeley, M.D.*, London, p. 73. Stukeley had been a medical student and colleague of Stephen Hales at Cambridge from 1703–1706. He was an eager dissector of animals: 'my Tutor gave me a room in the College to dissect in & practise chymical Experiments ... the wall was generally hung with Guts, stomachs, bladders ... . Here I and my Associats often dind upon the same table as our dogs lay upon', p. 33. As early as 1707 he had attended a Mr George Rolfe's anatomy lectures in London.

6 *Idem.*, p. 73. The College of Physicians had tried unsuccessfully for three years to obtain access to more executed bodies. They faced stiff opposition not only from the hanged person's family but from private anatomy lecturers and hospitals, who would pay the Sheriff far more to obtain possession of the body at the gallows than the College was willing. Stukeley appears to have attended the second reading of the bill in committee of the House of Lords. The bill failed and the College ceased to obtain bodies from Tyburn by the 1730s. On the scuffles that took place see Linebaugh, Peter (1975), 'The Tyburn Riot Against the Surgeons', in Douglas Hay, et al. (eds), *Albion's Fatal Tree: Crime and Society in Eighteenth-Century England*, New York: Pantheon Books, pp. 65–117.

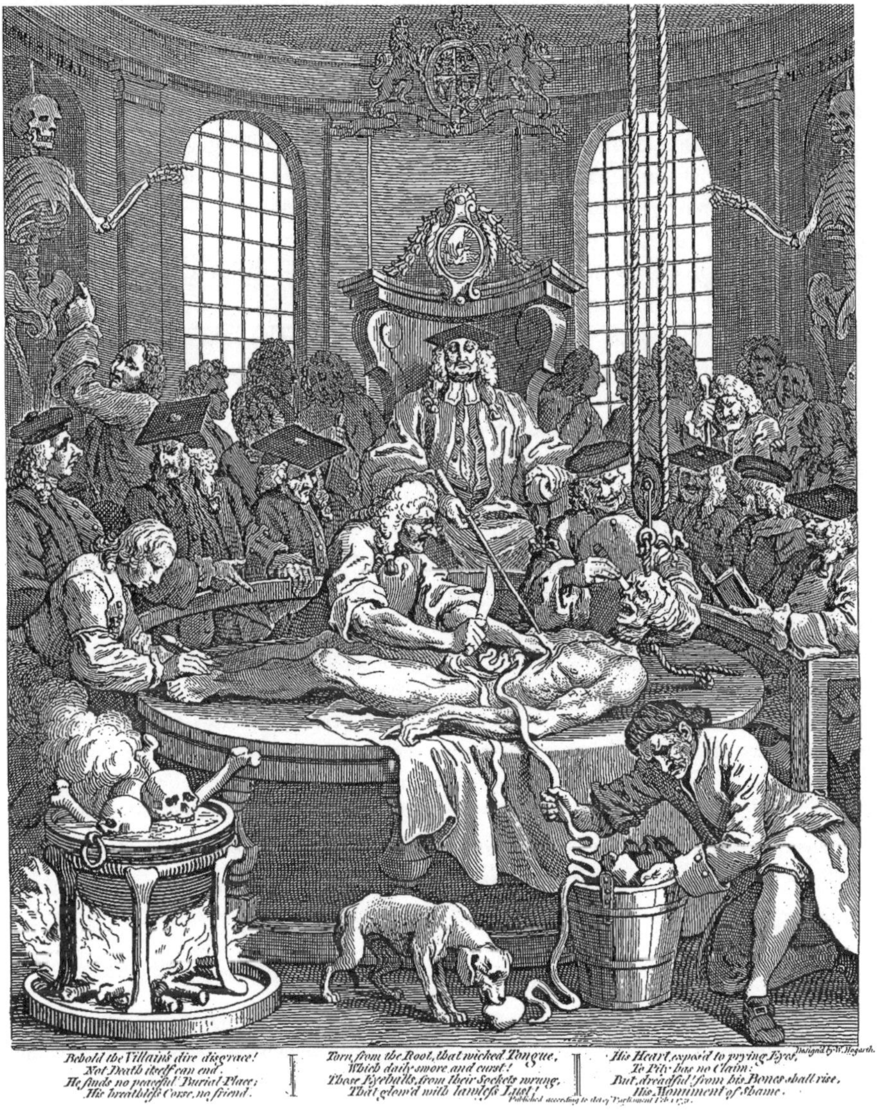
Behold the Villain's dire disgrace!
Not Death itself can end.
He finds no peaceful Burial-Place;
His breathless Corse, no friend.
Torn from the Root, that wicked Tongue,
Which daily swore and curst!
Those Eyeballs, from their Sockets wrung,
That glow'd with lawless Lust!
His Heart, expos'd to prying Eyes,
To Pity has no Claim:
But, dreadful! from his Bones shall rise,
His Monument of Shame.
Design'd by W. Hogarth.

Figure 6.1 William Hogarth, *The Reward of Cruelty*, 1751. The Wellcome Library, London.

rise in the mid eighteenth century.[7] Ruth Richardson sees the Murder Act as one of the many steps toward the commodification of the corpse among the ruling classes, an argument that seems borne out if the debates of the House of Lords in 1724 are compared to those of 1752.[8]

Under the terms of the Murder Act the body of the hanged was returned to Newgate Prison. From there it was transported a few yards to the building of the Surgeon's Company in the Old Bailey where dissection as a 'further Terror and peculiar mark of Infamy', was meant to be carried out.[9]

In fact, to satisfy the letter of the law following the stripping of the body of clothing by the hangman and the removal of the rope, a scalpel was briefly plunged into the chest of the corpse in front of the City Marshal. The hangman left to exhibit the clothing and rope at a local public house at so much per head. The body was then sewn up and sold to the highest bidder from an anatomy school in London.[10] So much for the legal sale of bodies. The question is where did anatomy teachers such as John and William Hunter – who literally required hundreds of corpses a year to keep their businesses going –actually obtain them? They turned to illegal means.

Illegal exhumation for dissection dates back to at least the seventeenth century in England. Initially the system of acquiring corpses was neither well organised nor was the scale of the operation large. Mostly it was dissection-room staff, graveyard labourers, medical students and teachers who indulged in bodysnatching from pauper cemeteries at night. It was even rumoured that in the early eighteenth century you could pay for your MD at Edinburgh University by supplying corpses to your teachers. Resurrecting was hard physical labour and sometimes medical students sought to avoid all that digging by bribing servants to gain access to the coffin of a dead master or mistress lying-in-state at home. The corpse would be replaced with weights and the coffin nailed down to avoid detection. This was a difficult feat to pull off as professional mourners were often employed to watch the body. There are very

---

7 Richardson, Ruth (2001), *Death, Dissection and the Destitute*, Chicago: University of Chicago Press, p. 35.

8 The 1832 Anatomy Act repealed the section of the 1752 Murder Act that pertained to dissection. From 1832 the Court could only order a body to be hung in chains or buried within the prison precincts. The penalty for violating the Anatomy Act was fixed at not more than three months imprisonment or a fine of £50. See *Anno secundo & tertio Gulielmi IV. Regis. Cap. LXXV. An Act for regulating Schools of Anatomy, 1st August 1832, section XVI.*

9 From 1796 the bodies were transported to the new hall of the Surgeon's Corporation in Lincoln's Inn Fields. See Blake, James Bailey (ed.) (1896), *The Diary of A Resurrectionist 1811–12*, London, p. 24.

10 Blake, p. 29. 'The Four Stages of Cruelty' were not popular prints like 'Gin Lane' and 'Beer Street' that were priced at one shilling each. Tom Nero's cap and the badge lettered 'St. G' identify him as a child in the care of the parish of St Giles-in-the-Fields, just to the west of Bloomsbury and one of the poorest and most notorious districts. Hogarth claimed the prints were 'calculated to reform some reigning vices peculiar to the lower class of people'. Reward of Cruelty Hall has been identified as the Cutlerian Theatre of the Royal College of Physicians in Warwick Lane, near Newgate, which the Surgeons' Company used from 1745–52 after separating from the old Barber-Surgeons' Company.

few descriptions of bodysnatching by medical students to be found in lecture notes or published works, perhaps because they were something to boast of in private:

> August 13 1761 at 7 o Clock in the morning, the surgeon lads carried off the Body of a Melancholique fellow, about 30, who had cut his throat the night before in several places with a Razor – The Body of this unhappy wretch was conveyed to Dr. Gregory's Laboratory in the Old Town and where Dr David thence performed the Dissection, and gave the following Lectures. L.1. The Trachea is cut immed.ly below the Cartilage ... .[11]

Even with the Murder Act of 1752 the Hunters, like other anatomy teachers, had to rely on the services of bodysnatchers, also known as resurrectionists, sack-em-up men or ghouls.

The key to a successful resurrection was speed and silence. Bodysnatchers surveyed graveyards ahead of time for possible escape routes and bribed sextons and grave diggers. Poor graveyards were generally targeted more than ones where the rich were buried because the graves of the poor were not very deep and often a pauper grave yielded three or four bodies stacked one on top of the other.[12] Robert Christison, a house-surgeon at the Edinburgh Infirmary from 1818 to 1820, gave a detailed description of bodysnatching in his memoirs:

> The resurrectionists in Edinburgh were chiefly assistants of the several teachers of anatomy ... . A hole was dug down to the coffin only where the head lay – a canvas sheet being stretched around to receive the earth, and to prevent any of it spoiling the smooth uniformity of the grass. The digging was done with short, flat, dagger-shaped implements of wood, to avoid the clicking noise of iron striking stones. On reaching the coffin, two broad iron hooks under the lid, pulled forcibly up with a rope, broke off a sufficient portion of the lid to allow the body to be dragged out; and sacking was heaped over the whole to deaden the sound of the cracking wood. The body was stripped of the grave-clothes, which were scrupulously buried again; it was secured in a sack; and the surface of the ground was carefully restored to its original condition, – which was not difficult, as the sod over a fresh-filled grave must always present signs of recent disturbance. The whole process could be completed in an hour, even though the grave might be six feet deep, because the soil was loose, and the digging was done impetuously by frequent relays of active men. Transference over the churchyard wall was easy in a dark evening; and once in the street, the carrier of the sack drew no attention at so early an hour.[13]

Christison remarked that country churchyards were chosen for the convenience of approach and their distance from houses. The body was stripped and taken naked for, under both English and Scottish law, it was a felony to steal the shroud or any clothing, but only a misdemeanour to take the body itself because no one could own

---

11 Anonymous (1761), *Dr. David, 2 lectures on dissection*, f. 1, College of Physicians of Philadelphia, uncatalogued manuscript. It is likely from the reference to Dr Gregory and the Old Town, that this took place in Edinburgh, but one cannot be sure.

12 For example there are numerous references to bodies being stolen in the Vestry Minutes of the Westminster City Archives and *Lloyd's Evening Post* and the *British Chronicle* from the 1760s on. I thank Elaine Reynolds for providing these.

13 Christison, Robert (1885), *The Life of Robert Christison,* London, edited by his sons, p. 176.

a body. The only charge that could be brought against those who stole a naked body was trespass.[14]

The Times reported many cases of bodysnatching. Typical was the following:

> On Monday evening, a set of Resurrectionists, were apprehended at a house near the Turnpike, Mile End. That morning a coach was observed to stop at this house, and an ill-looking fellow came out of it with a sack, containing as was supposed, a body, which he carried into the house and returned immediately with a large hamper; they then drove off to a neighbouring public-house, when after a short stay they took up some others and were traced to the Launch, at Deptford. In the mean time the Parish Officers were informed of the circumstance. About 6 in the evening the coach again returned with a similar lading, which was deposited in the house. Some constables accompanied by a number of people surrounded the house, and forcing an entrance, they found 2 men and a woman, drinking tea on a bench, at one end of which lay the bodies of 2 children. They were secured; 6 adults were discovered unmutilated, besides which the floor was strewed with limbs in a state too shocking for public description.[15]

Charles Nicholas Jenty, a man-midwife and anatomy and surgery lecturer in London, addressed the stories of medical students stealing corpses for teaching purposes in the preface to *A Course of Anatomico-Physiological Lectures on the Human Structure and Animal Oeconomy* (1757). 'Witness the Story of MEDEA, who was branded with the Inhumanity of boiling Men alive, for no other Reason, but because she invented warm Baths. And who, to this Day, can persuade the Vulgar, but the Pupils of anatomical Schools secretly convey People in order to dissect them?'[16] Unfortunately proclaiming it was all just a misunderstanding with Medea was not enough to dispel the rumours.

As public awareness of the wide scope of bodysnatching started to grow, anatomists, fearful of riots outside their schools, turned to offering money for corpses rather than snatching them themselves.[17] By the early nineteenth century resurrecting had become a lucrative profession for gangs who, on occasion, attacked each other in graveyards and broke into dissecting rooms to mutilate bodies acquired by other gangs for anatomy teachers.[18] At a Parliamentary Inquiry in 1828 into the

14 See Ross, Ian and Ross, Carol Urquhart, (1980), 'Body Snatching in Nineteenth Century Britain: From Exhumation to Murder', *British Journal of Law and Society*, 6 (1), pp. 108–18. The authors state that in 1644 the principle of the legal recognition of no property in a body (caro data vermibus [is] nullius in bonis) was established. The King's Bench case of Rex v Lynn in 1788 further developed the principle. Lynn was charged with disinterring a corpse for the purposes of dissection. The Court ruled that bodysnatching did not constitute theft and merely fined Lynn.

15 *The Times*, Thursday 20 March 1794, p. 3.

16 Jenty, Charles Nicholas (1757), *A Course of Anatomico-Physiological Lectures on the Human Structure and Animal Oeconomy*, London, p. xxxi.

17 There were riots in Scotland, Dublin and Oxford in the 1770s.

18 See Richardson, Chapter Five. Also Durey, M.J. (1976), 'Body snatchers and Benthamites: The Implications of the Dead Body Bill for the London Schools of Anatomy, 1820–42', *The London Journal*, 2 (2), pp. 200–25, and Knott, John (1985), 'Popular Attitudes to Death and Dissection in Early Nineteenth Century Britain: The Anatomy Act and the Poor',

illegal supply of bodies to anatomy schools and hospitals, Joshua Brookes, a surgeon and teacher, was called to give evidence. The Inquiry would eventually result in the passing of the Anatomy Act in 1832, which made it legal for medical men to take unclaimed bodies from hospitals and workhouses. Brookes had been trained by former students of the Hunters and he described several instances of difficulties in working with resurrectionists to obtain subjects for his anatomy school: bodies delivered in the evening were stolen back in the middle of the night to be resold to another teacher who would pay more for them; one of his 'subjects' was cut to pieces in his dissecting-room by a rival gang of bodysnatchers who waved knives in the faces of the students when they tried to seize the body back; and when Brookes failed to agree to pay more for his teaching materials, the gang he used left two decomposing bodies outside his front door at dusk that a pair of nicely dressed young ladies stumbled over. This, Joshua Brookes solemnly told the Parliamentary Select Committee, had brought unwelcome publicity to his anatomy school.[19]

In anonymous evidence to the Select Committee in 1828, Ben Crouch – leader of the most notorious gang in London from 1800 to 1825 – estimated that there were between 40 and 50 full-time resurrectionists in London. He boasted that he had personally dug up 23 bodies from one cemetery over the course of four nights and sold them to three different anatomy teachers. Joseph Naples, another bodysnatcher questioned by the Committee, read from his account book in which he listed all the bodies his gang provided to anatomy teachers in the capital from 1800 to 1825. Part of this book has miraculously survived and is in the collections of the Royal College of Surgeons in London.[20] According to the scribbled notes, in 1809, Naples was responsible for 305 adults and 44 small subjects under three feet being dug up and sold to various schools. Thirty-seven more were exported to Edinburgh and 18 subjects on hand were never used. The adults cost four guineas on average while the 'smalls' (children) were sold at six shillings for the first foot and nine pence an inch after that.[21]

The Hunters enter this scenario during an intermediary phase after the time when anatomists had to supply their own raw material and before they delegated this responsibility to the gangs.[22] There is evidence to suggest that the brothers both liaised with, and perhaps served as resurrectionists.

Labour History (Canberra) 49, pp. 1–18. On bodysnatchers breaking into the dissecting room at St Thomas' Hospital and menacing the students with knives to get paid for delivery of corpses see (1825), *An Account of the Circumstances Attending the Imprisonment and Death of the late William Millard, London, printed and pub. by Ann Millard*, p. 16.

19 *Report From The Select Committee on Anatomy, Ordered by the House of Commons to be Printed, 22 July 1828.*

20 Sixteen pages of the *Diary* remain from 1811–12. Notes at the Royal College of Surgeons indicate that a dresser to Mr Bransby Cooper bought the diary from a person who had supplied bodies to dissecting rooms.

21 (1811–12), *The Diary of A Resurrectionist*, Royal College of Surgeons, MS. 67/a.5.

22 Richardson, Chapter Five.

The Hunters and the body trade

As the young James Williams discovered while a pupil lodging with William Hunter, human bodies were bought and sold like any other commodity. Besides stealing fresh bodies from graveyards, private homes and workhouse death-rooms (mortuaries), salted and pickled cadavers were imported by London anatomy teachers from as far away as Holy Fields Hospital in Dublin and the large charity hospitals of Paris. In the 1750s John Hunter was chiefly responsible for procuring corpses for his brother's school:

> ... he went by the familiar title of 'Jack Hunter'[and] was employed by his brother to cater for the dissecting-room, in the course of which employment he became a great favourite with that certainly not too respectable class of persons the resurrection men ... .[23]

By the 1770s John Hunter was purchasing bodies and preparations to add to the growing collection of rarities which he kept at his large house and museum in Leicester Square and at his country cottage and zoo in the village of Earls Court. At the former he taught students anatomy and surgery. They no doubt marvelled at the stuffed cameoleopard, or giraffe, which graced the front hallway. John Hunter craved anatomical rarities:

> He was indeed a most resolute beggar for every specimen which particularly pleased him by its rarity, and which chanced to be in the possession of any of his friends. The late Dr. Clarke had a preparation of an extra-uterine pregnancy, in which the foetus had been detained in the fallopian tube, and had there undergone partial development, when the mother died from internal haemorrhage, consequent on the rupture of the tube. On this specimen he set a high value, and Hunter had often viewed it with longing eyes. 'Come, Doctor,' said he, 'I positively must have that preparation.' 'No, John Hunter,' was the reply, 'You positively shall not.' 'You will not give it me, then?' 'No.' 'Will you sell it?' 'No.' 'Well then, take care I don't meet you with it in some dark lane at night, for if I do, I'll murder you to get it.'[24]

John Hunter wrote to one of his favourite students, Edward Jenner of vaccination fame, in 1786 and asked him to scout out the chances of stealing a specimen. However, he was cautious in asking Jenner to confirm that it was worth taking:

> I am told there is the skin of a toad in Berkeley Castle that is of prodigious size. Let me know the truth of it, its dimensions, what bones are still in it, and if it can be stolen by some invisible being.[25]

We have no evidence that he obtained the toad.

In 1783 John Hunter obtained his most famous specimen – the body of Charles O'Byrne, the Irish Giant. Born in 1761 at Littlebridge in Ireland, O'Byrne's parents were of normal size but reportedly had conceived their son on top of a tall haystack and this had led to his excessive height. In 1782 he was first exhibited in a shop in

---

23 Ottley, Drewry (1835), *The Life of John Hunter*, London, p. 10.

24 Ibid., p. 75.

25 Ibid., p. 104.

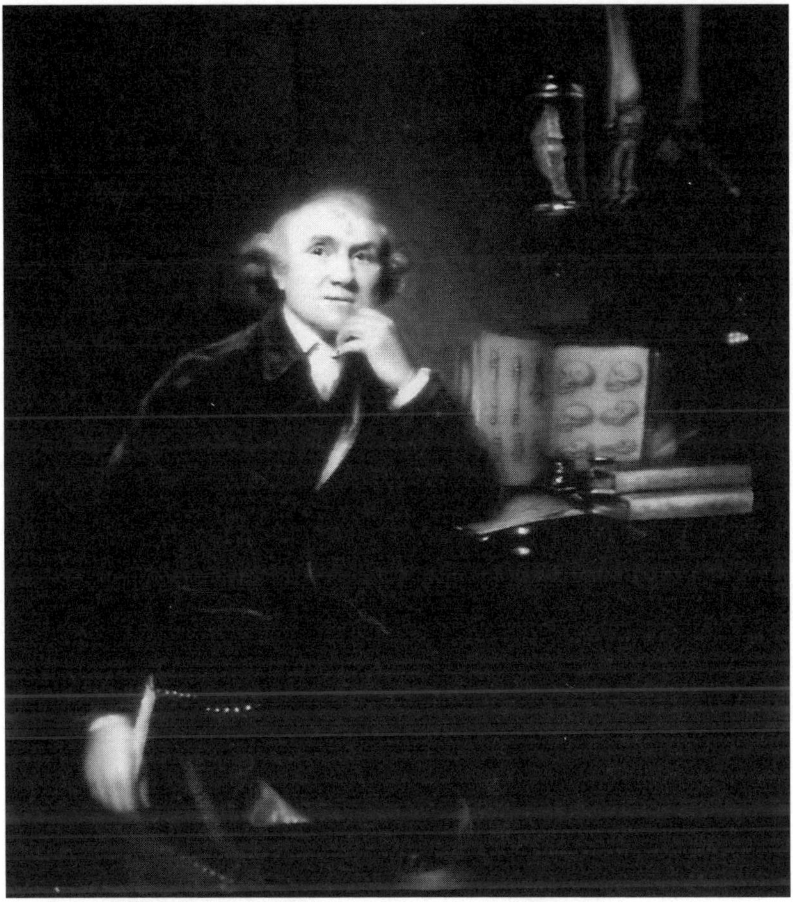

Figure 6.2 ***John Hunter*** **by Sir Joshua Reynolds, 1786. By kind permission of the Royal College of Surgeons of England.**

London as, 'Mr. Byrne, the surprising Irish Giant, who is allowed to be the tallest man in the world; only 21 years of age ...'[26] A year later, O'Byrne completed a tour of the British Isles where he entertained the public by lighting his pipe from street lamps. He returned very sick to London. Among many others, Hunter had the house watched where Byrne lay dying, blind and demented from a probable brain tumour and alcoholism. The *Morning Herald* reported on 5 June 1783 that:

> The whole tribe of surgeons put in a claim for the poor departed Irish Giant and surrounded his house just as Greenland harpooners would an enormous whale.[27]

26 Dobson, Jesse (1953), 'Observables at the Royal College of Surgeons. 42. Charles Byrne: The Irish Giant', *Annals of the Royal College of Surgeons of England*, 13 (1), July, pp. 63–5. Quotation from p. 63.

27 Ibid., p. 65.

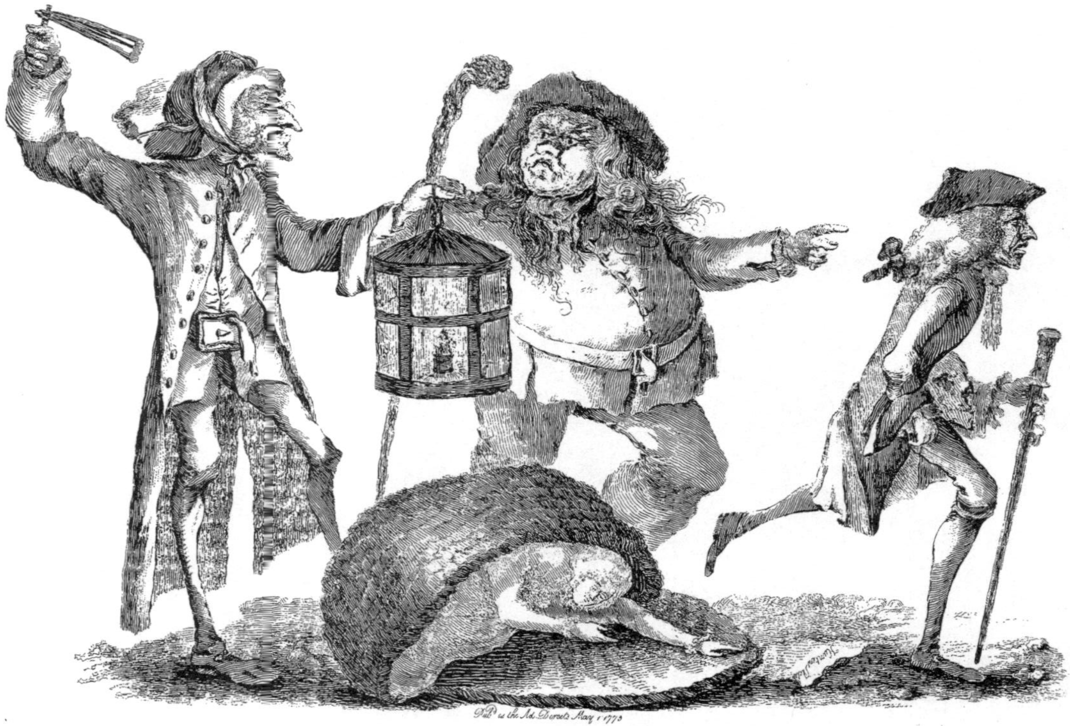

Figure 6.3 *The anatomist overtaken by the watch in carrying off Miss W--ts in a hamper*. **Etching with engraving by W. Austin, 1773. The Wellcome Library, London.**

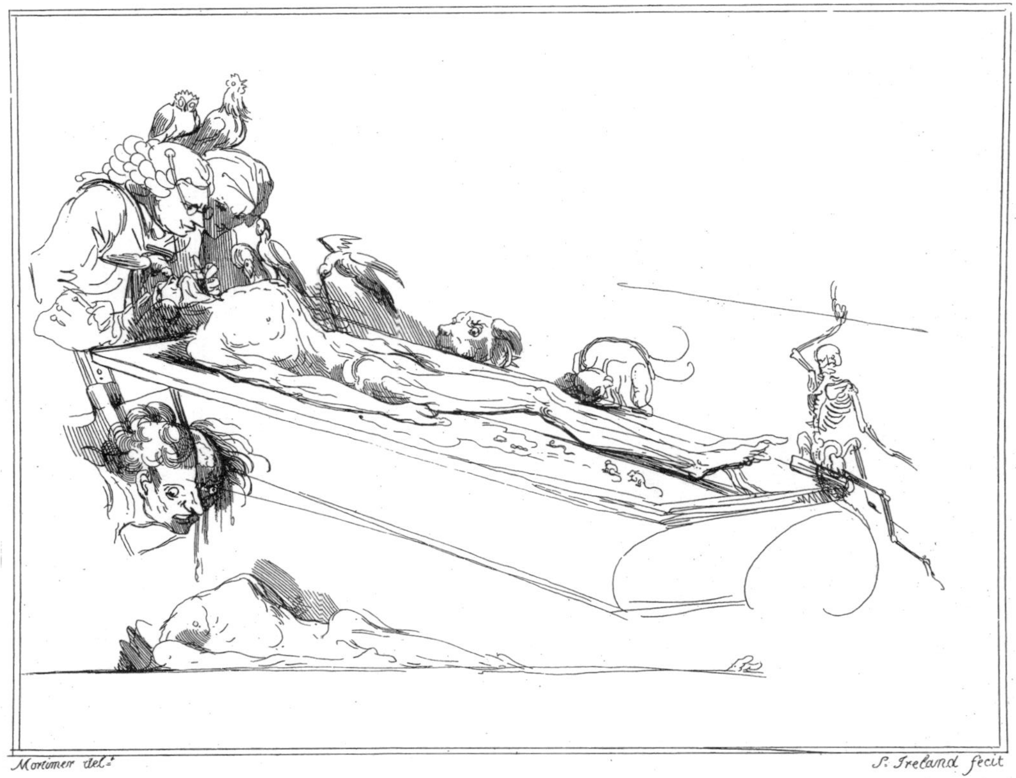

Figure 6.4 **Anonymous, *Two anatomists dissecting a corpse, surrounded by birds, a cat, a dog and mice*. Etching by S. Ireland after a drawing by J.H. Mortimer, eighteenth century. The Wellcome Library, London.**

In the knowledge that John Hunter and other anatomy teachers wanted his body for a specimen, Charles O'Byrne, begged his friends to bury him at sea in a lead coffin. He died on 1 June 1783. Hunter found out which public house the watchers of the body were drinking in as the coffin was being made. He bribed the undertaker with 50 pounds if he would agree to the body being 'kidnapped' as it travelled from London to Margate. John was renowned for his lack of financial sense, unlike his brother William who died a millionaire. The eventual price for the corpse of the poor giant was a staggering 500 pounds – which Hunter had to borrow from a friend.

Hunter had the body transported by hackney coach to his country place in Earl's Court while the Giant's so-called friends placed paving stones in the coffin and buried it at sea. Hunter was concerned that the theft of such a famous corpse would be quickly publicized, and instead of a leisurely dissection, he sliced the body up and dropped it into a huge copper boiler to strip the flesh from the bones quickly. As a result the skeleton was, and is, brown. John Hunter was immensely proud of having snatched the body of the giant, and he even had part of the skeleton (the feet) included in a 1786 painting of himself by Joshua Reynolds.

What of the bodysnatching activities of William Hunter? Horace Walpole referred to 'Dr. Hunter, that Scotch night man' in a letter to the Reverend William Mason. Walpole was upset that Hunter's politics had shifted from his party to the royal family with Hunter's appointment as accoucheur.[28] Yet the choice of the insult of 'night man' is interesting, as an engraving of 1773 by W. Austin shows William Hunter as a bodysnatcher. Hunter is depicted making off with a skull under his arm as a night watchman, carrying a large lantern, seizes a body snatcher. A female corpse falls out of a hamper. Hunter is identified in the engraving by the paper he has dropped. It reads 'Hunter's lec[res].'

A second image likens the two anatomists hovering over the head of the corpse to the birds of prey which are shown pecking at it. The owl that perches on one of the dissectors is the attribute of Athena (the goddess of wisdom), while the rooster on that of his companion is Aesculapius' attribute (the god of medicine). Possibly the first anatomist is William Hunter and the second is John Hunter, with the rooster being a reference to his experiments regarding transplanting human teeth into a cockscomb, or does it refer to his lack of modesty when it came to crowing his successes?[29] The birds, cats, dogs and mice further extend the image of predators and prey.

The ibis is an Egyptian vulture and this label for William Hunter may have originated from the ill feeling that the artist Jan van Rymsdyck held for him. Rymsdyck provided 34 of the drawings for Hunter's *The Anatomy of the Human Gravid Uterus*

28 Simmons, p. 55.

29 The dissected rooster's head with the human tooth in place is still on display at the Hunterian Museum at the Royal College of Surgeons in London, as is the poor giant's brown skeleton.

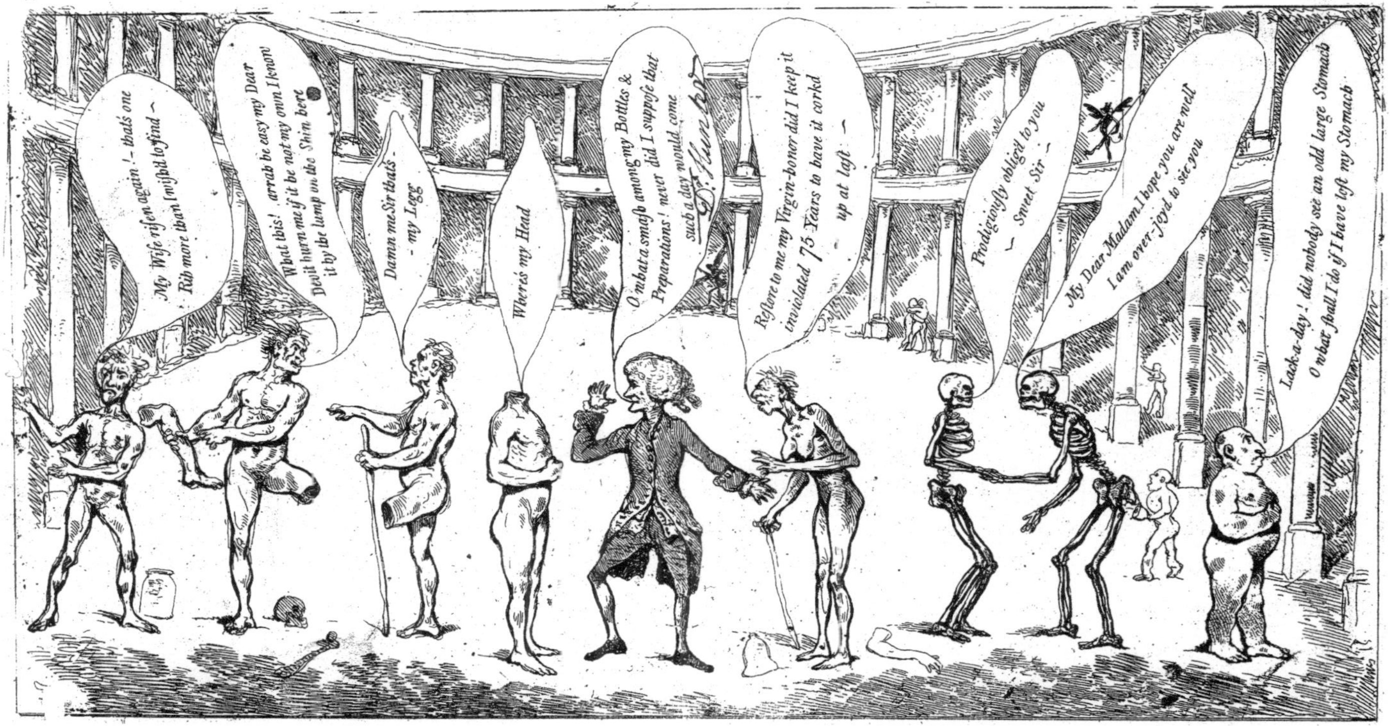
My Wife risen again ! – that's one Rib more than I wish'd to find –
What this ! arrah be easy my Dear Devil burn me if it be not my own I know it by the lump on the Shin here
Damn me Sir thats – my Legg
Where's my Head
O what a smash among my Bottles & Preparations ! never did I suppose that such a day would come
Dr. Hunter
Restore to me my Virgin-honor did I keep it inviolated 75 Years to have it cork'd up at last –
Prodigiously oblig'd to you – Sweet Sir –
My Dear Madam I hope you are well I am over-joy'd to see you
Lack-a-day ! did nobody see an odd large Stomach O what shall I do if I have lost my Stomach

Figure 6.5 Anonymous, ***The Resurrection or an internal View of the Museum in W--d-m-ll Street on the last Day***, **1782. The Wellcome Library, London.**

(1774).[30] In the preface to the atlas Hunter praised the skill of the French engraver but not that of Rymsdyk. Partly in revenge Rymsdyk published a book in 1778, titled *Museum Brittanicum: An Exhibition of a Great Variety of Antiquities and Curiousities Belonging to that Noble and Magnificent Cabinet, the British Museum.* Despite its long title this was a small volume with 30 mediocre plates, drawn by his son, and huge footnotes written by the senior Rymsdyk criticizing just about everything and everybody. In a footnote that starts on page four and continues to page seven, Rymsdyck savaged the Royal Academy of Arts (where William Hunter was Professor of Anatomy) and denounced a series of characters who persecuted him. They included:

> ... the Stiff Clergyman; Double-fee Lawyers; Dr. Last, the physician; Dr. Grooper, the Man-Midwife, the Churchyard Shark, or Anatomist who will make a skeleton of your Deceased Wife etc. after You have been to the expense of 100 l. or 200 l. in keeping her alive and bestowing a decent burial upon the Corpse ... .[31]

This veiled reference to Mrs Van Butchell was followed by a discussion of birds and their eggs in the British Museum including:

> ... the Ibis, 'hieroglyphic of Mercury, god of messengers and thieves, alike, and of medicine'. The Ibis, a bird common in Egypt 'with a long hooked bill of a fine red, long stiff legs, and the colour of its feathers all over of a shining black', is worshipped by the Egyptians as a god.[32]

Rymsdyk then refers to a famous anatomist and bodysnatcher who perfectly matches this description, a Dr Ibis, 'who ill-used and betrayed him'.[33]

A final example of the public perception of the Hunters as bodysnatchers comes from an anonymous engraving. William Hunter is portrayed fully clothed, standing in his spacious, classically inspired museum. He is surrounded by his living anatomies and various preparations.[34] He appears far more concerned with his inanimate and priceless preparations than the hapless resurrected corpses who

---

30 Jordanova Ludmilla (1985), 'Gender, generation and science: William Hunter's obstetrical atlas', in Bynum, William and Porter, Roy (eds), *William Hunter and the Eighteenth Century Medical World*, Cambridge and New York: Cambridge University Press, p. 390.

31 Corner, Betsy Copping (1951), 'Dr. Ibis and the Artists: A Sidelight upon Hunter's Atlas, *The Gravid Uterus*', *Journal of the History of Medicine and Allied Sciences*, 1, pp. 1–21. Quotation from p. 14.

32 Corner, p. 18.

33 *Idem.*

34 Susan Lawrence describes the museum in (1995), 'Anatomy and Address Creating Medical Gentlemen in Eighteenth-Century London', Nutton, Vivian and Porter, Roy (eds), *The History of Medical Education in Britain*, Amsterdam: Rodolphi Press, p. 211. Simmons, in (1784), *Two Introductory Lectures, delivered by William Hunter, to his last course of Anatomical Lectures, at his Theatre in Windmill-Street: As they were left corrected for the Press by himself. Printed by order of the Trustees, for J. Johnson*, London, described the museum as a 'magnificent room fitted up with great elegance and propriety.' p. 57. F.J. Cole states that between 1739 and 1800, 39 anatomical museums were founded in England. (1914), *History of the Anatomical Museum*, London, p. 305.

plaintively clutch amputated limbs, for he exclaims 'Oh what a smash among my Bottles & Preparations! Never did I suppose that such a day would come.' Perhaps this was a reference to Hunter's own day of judgement for performing dissections so indiscriminately on these doubly resurrected bodies. Littered around the floor are limbs, organs and skulls, missing from the hapless victims who profess such witticisms as 'where's my head?' to fighting words over 'whose leg is that?' and finally 'Restore to me my Virgin-honour did I keep it inviolated 75 years to have it corked up at last.' Such black humour reflected the deep-seated fear of being snatched from the grave by Hunter's paid gangs and the religious consequences of going to meet one's Maker in pieces. This would deny the Christian sentiment for permitting the undisturbed natural decay of the integral body and the belief in the physical resurrection on the Day of Judgement of the whole body.[35]

What do these images tell us about medical dispassion? Certainly both Hunters seem to have overcome any sentimental feelings about purchasing bodies or parts. William appears to have had John do the dirty work (literally) but it is interesting that there are no known etchings or engravings of John as a bodysnatcher. Is this because John was blatant about buying specimens and William's secrecy made him a better target for satire? After all, John had Joshua Reynolds include the Irish Giant's feet in his self-portrait. Or was it because of William's money and gentlemanly manners? There are some common values in the images – avarice, glee and dedication to the activity of seeing and owning knowledge of the body. All of these values are captured in a watercolour done by Thomas Rowlandson, in about1780, traditionally identified as the dissecting room at the Great Windmill Street Anatomy School.[36] It was beneath this attic that the young James Williams tried to sleep despite the stench emanating from John Hunter's preparations next door and the swearing of the resurrectionists as they heaved bodies up the stairs to the attic.

Rowlandson portrayed dissecting as a veritable feeding frenzy. William Hunter is shown supervising from on high in a room decorated with animal and human

35 See Richardson, pp. 3–29 and pp. 75–99.

36 The description of the lithograph in the online catalogue of the Wellcome Library notes that Dr Helen Brock questioned whether this could be Hunter's dissecting room in Windmill Street, as dissections took place underneath the anatomy theatre, so the skylight makes little sense. The Wellcome Library, however, concludes that 'The Rowlandson caricature probably depicts the dissecting room at Windmill Street.' But as shown in Chapter Five, in his first lecture, William Hunter discussed the light and seating in his theatre and why that meant the cadaver could be best viewed at his lectures rather than at rival schools. '[A] strong sky-light is thrown upon the table, and the glass being ground, that is, made rough upon one surface, the glare of sun-shine is not admitted.' We know that John Hunter's anatomy theatre at his home in Leicester Square was similarly lit – for obvious reasons anatomists did not want windows that people could see through, nor did they want heat from the sun speeding the decay of the body. See the ground plan drawn by William Clift in 1832 of the Leicester Square residence. Clift drew it from memory 'as it was in the year 1792'. He labelled each part of the house including 'Where Mr Huger met the Irishman'. Huger was a house pupil and no doubt received delivery of O'Byrne's body. The original plan is among the Clift papers at the Royal College of Surgeons and a copy made by Fenwick Beekman in 1936 is in the New York Academy of Medicine.

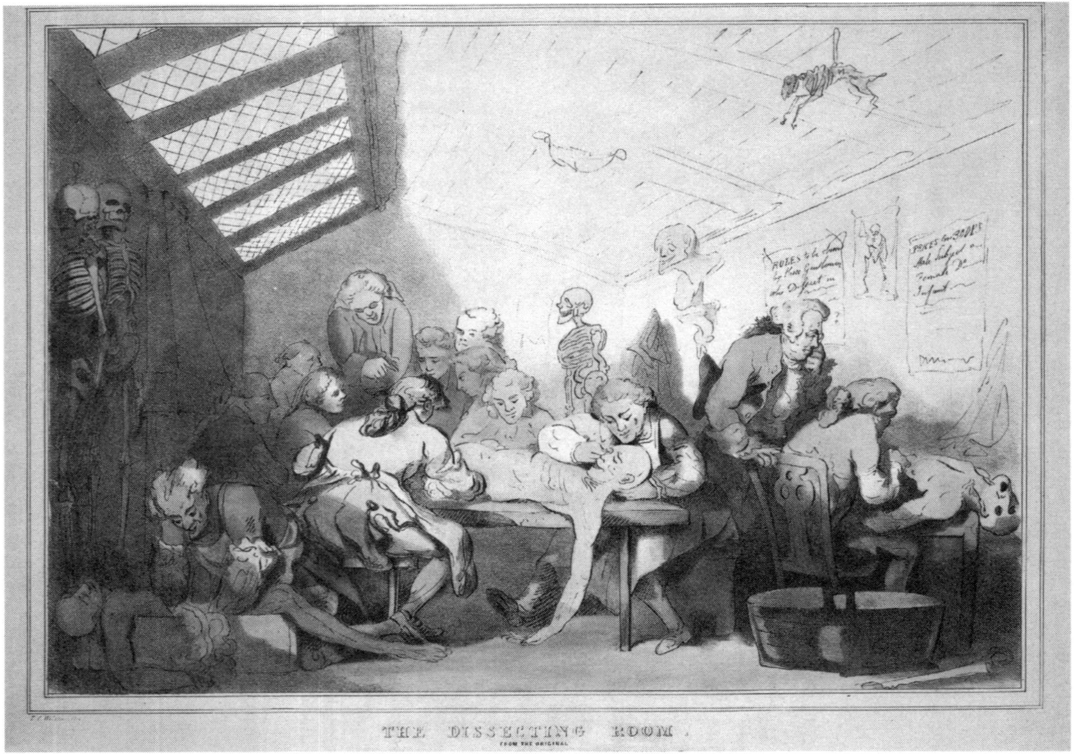

Figure 6.6 **Coloured lithograph by T.C. Wilson after a pen and wash drawing by T. Rowlandson of *The Dissecting Room*, *c.*1780. The Wellcome Library, London.**

skeletons. Along the right wall can be glimpsed a list of rules on how to conduct oneself when dissecting. As discussed earlier, William Hunter, in fact, had his rules hanging on the wall of the dissection room. Three naked corpses are in various stages of being cut up and young men huddle around them. Several of them have been identified, including John Hunter, Tobias Smollett, Matthew Baillie, William Cruikshank, John Howison, David Pitcairn, John Sheldon and Pierre Camper. All were students of William Hunter at various different times making this picture a fantasy one. The corpses are limp and cooperative, no books are in evidence and instruments and fingers greedily disembowel a body and dissect an eye while leering skeletons watch. Here are the Hunters with their club of pupils raptly poking, prodding and slicing up three corpses in gleeful camaraderie. One might say that they are shown being passionate about being dispassionate enough to dissect. They also appear not to have a care in the world, but we know from lectures by William Hunter that dissecting did not come easy and we know from lectures by William Cruikshank that the dissecting room was not the most pleasant place on earth.

Cruikshank noticed that the students at the Great Windmill Street School 'were seized with *diarrhœa*, as soon as they began their dissecting'. He believed this was due to 'swallowing the putrid effluvia along with the saliva'.[37] In other words the stench of the decaying bodies made them sick. Cruikshank continued that 'with time the constitution becomes gradually accustomed to the infectious effluvia.' It does not seem to have occurred to him that diarrhoea could have been from horror and disgust at cutting rancid bodies open. Cruikshank checked with his counterpart, Henry Cline, at St Thomas' Hospital and discovered that his new students also frequently had diarrhoea. He wondered if it was due to the cold in the dissecting room, but Cline told him that they had a huge fire burning in their dissecting room. This must have made the bodies smell even worse. Cruikshank was forced to conclude, contrary to William Hunter, that dead bodies could be infectious.[38] What to do?

> I am not aware, that giving a contrary opinion, in public, can deter students from their duty; or make them more afraid of looking into the dead body. We all know that fevers may be caught at hospitals, from the living body; yet physicians do not complain of want of pupils; and he would be reckoned a sorry student, who would not do his duty at the risk of his health .... Besides the authority of the anatomist will be insufficient to convince the pupil of the inoffensive nature of putrid vapour, whilst he feels his own nature revolt at it, and his other preceptors in medicine maintain a contrary doctrine.[39]

This was Cruikshank in 1779, four years before William Hunter died and named him and Baillie as partners in the Anatomy School.

If we now turn to Cruikshank's lectures nearly 20 years later, it appears that he did everything possible to convince his students that any sickness they experienced on entering the dissecting room was due to the cold of the place:

---

37 Clare, P. (1779), *An Essay on the Cure of Abscesses by Caustic*, London. Clare was a surgeon at Barts and Cruikshank's remarks appear in the Appendix under the title of 'Remarks on the New Method of introducing Mercury into the Circulation' p. 117.

38 Clare, pp. 117–18.

39 Ibid., p. 120.

> Anatomists in general have liv'd to a great age – do not believe there is anything pernicious to health in the air of a dissecting room, or in dissecting unless you cut yourself, and then it is very unfrequently anything disagreeable happens unless the body has died of a putrid fever or venereal compli[cations] etc – Catarrh and Diarhoea are frequently got in dissecting but this is unconnected with the dead body as it is from the necessary cold of the place: would therefore recommend the use of fleecy Hosiery.[40]

This was a debate that would continue well into the nineteenth century. But Cruikshank appears to have recognized that his timid charges needed reassurance that getting sick when first dissecting was not due to their tender natures but due to the temperature of the dissecting room – or if you were unlucky enough to cut yourself. The Hunters had taught him that the heart of an anatomy school was its dissecting room and it was there that boys were made into medical men.

John Hunter as teacher and surgeon

> When Mr. Physick brought his son as a new pupil, and asked what books he should read, Hunter said, 'Sir follow me; I will show you the books your son has to study'; took him into the dissecting room and showed him the bodies; 'these are the books your son will learn under my direction, the others are fit for very little.[41]

John Hunter began his course of lectures on surgery with the proud statement that, 'I am to deliver nothing that I have not seen and observed myself, I am not a reader of Books.'[42] He then explained why books were of little use to the medical man:

> Too much attention cannot be paid to the structure & situation of the human body. This knowledge will show the parts which can be cut etc. – .
> Books of surgery are mere lists of Operations and cases. The steps of an Operation are described; an account is given of the pulse, stools etc. Any porter of an Hospital may with a few months teaching compose such a Book.[43]

As mentioned elsewhere, John Hunter was appointed as a surgeon at St George's Hospital in 1754, a position he kept his entire life. After a stint as an army surgeon in the Seven Years War, he severed contact with his brother's school and opened a series

40 *Second Course – Saturday 20th January, 1798 Mr. Cruikshank, Introductory Lecture — On the Origins of Anatomy*. The Notes taken by William Clift, f. 12v.

41 Paget, p. 233. See also Jacyna, Stephen (1992), 'Physiological principles in the surgical writings of John Hunter', Lawrence, Christopher, *Medical Theory: Surgical Practice*, London: Routledge, pp. 135–152. He states that 'Given his concept of the organism as an intelligent entity that responded to injury in a remedial way, it is clear that Hunter did not regard the body as passive material upon which the surgeon must work according to his own lights. Rather, there had to be some attempt to harmonise the efforts of the healing art with the inherent curative power of nature.' p. 141.

42 John Hunter, (1790) *Lectures on Surgery* taken by Richard Stone, London, f. 168v, New York Academy of Medicine.

43 *Idem.*

of anatomy schools in London. There he taught practical anatomy, or dissecting and the preparation of specimens for medical teaching. In 1774 he gave his first course of lectures in surgery. Eventually there were 86 lectures in all. Whereas William was frightened of surgery, John was frightened of lecturing. In his biography of John Hunter in 1794 Jesse Foot claimed:

> His delivery was heavy and unengaging, as he rarely raised his eyes from his book; and as, in addition to this, the doctrines he taught were new, and often obscure and theoretical, his hearers were never numerous.[44]

This may have been due to the fact that John Hunter suffered from stage fright. According to Everard Home, one of John Hunter's pupils:

> ... he never commenced a course of lectures without having recourse to (30 drops of) laudanum to relieve his uneasy feelings, he notwithstanding continued the practice of lecturing for many years.[45]

John Hunter's lectures were never valued as highly as his brother's, perhaps due to his delivery of them in an opium-induced haze but also because he:

> Frequently changed his opinions and made notes that were unintelligible to him – even during lectures. Such a mode of lecturing was not likely to become popular; his class consequently never exceeded thirty, and not half that number derived much benefit from their attendance.[46]

Yet this is not to suggest that John Hunter's teaching was without impact. During his lifetime he instructed a thousand or more students in practical surgery at St George's Hospital. His strength lay in instructing students at the bedside of patients and in the dissecting room, rather than in the lecture room:

> In the Course of these Lectures I shall differ very much from what is taught in Books on the Subject of Surgery. The Ideas I have to communicate are mostly my own & not drawn from Books I have Reason to suppose them true because they are founded on Facts.[47]

While William desired students not to have read books, John was contemptuous of the books they had read. In both cases the Hunters represented that their lectures were not only superior to reading but were more truthful because they were based on a sustained programme of dissections and experiments taken from nature. John Hunter's most famous experiment was on himself. In *A Treatise on the Venereal Disease* (1786), Hunter described the following:

> To ascertain several facts relative to the venereal disease, the following experiments were made. They were begun in May 1767.

---

44 Ottley, p. 252.

45 *Idem*.

46 Ottley, p. 49.

47 Anonymous (1758), *John Hunters Lectures*, Wellcome Library, WMS/MSL40 a&b, f. 8.

> Two punctures were made on the penis with a lancet dipped in venereal matter from a gonnorhoea; one puncture was on the glans, the other on the prepuce.
> This was on a Friday; on the Sunday following there was a teasing itching in those parts which lasted till the Tuesday following. In the meantime these parts being often examined, there seemed to be a greater redness and moisture than usual, which was imputed to the parts being rubbed. Upon the Tuesday morning the parts of the prepuce where the puncture had been made were redder, thickened, and had formed a speck ... .[48]

Hunter observed that sores developed on the penis which he repeatedly touched with a caustic. Two months after treating a bubo (a swelling in a gland in the right groin) with mercury, an ulcer appeared on the tonsils:

> The mercury was thrown in by the same leg and thigh as before ... as soon as the ulcer was skinned over the mercury was left off, it not being intended to destroy the poison, but to observe what parts it would next affect. About three months after, copper coloured blotches broke out on the skin, and the former ulcer returned in the tonsil.[49]

Hunter applied mercury again – not to effect a cure – but to heal the ulcer so he could mark where it next occurred. As it simply reappeared in the same place, Hunter then gave enough mercury to produce a cure, 'The time the experiment took up, from the first insertion to the complete cure, was about three years.'[50] The penis in this experiment was John Hunter's.[51]

He found his hospital patients also offered opportunities for treatment and experimentation:

> A man had been afflicted with the venereal disease for a long time ... He was taken into St. George's Hospital, affected with a number of pocky sores; and before I put him under a mercurial course I made the following experiment: I took some matter from one of the sores upon the point of a lancet, and made three small wounds upon the back where the skin was smooth and sound, deep enough to draw blood. I made a wound similar to the other three, with a clean lancet, the four wounds making a quadrangle; but all the wounds healed up and none of them ever appeared after.
>
> This experiment I have repeated more than once, and with the same result; it shows that a pocky person cannot be affected locally with the matter proceeding from the sores produced by the lues venerea.[52]

---

48 See Hunter, John (1786), *A Treatise on the Venereal Disease,* p. 325 for details of this and of other experiments. Also see William Ashmead, *Physiological Lectures by John Hunter, F.R.S.*, London, 28 October 1777, College of Physicians of Philadelphia, MS 10a 165, for Hunter's experiments on patients with lues venera, f. 297v.

49 Hunter, *A Treatise on the Venereal Disease*, p. 326.

50 *Idem.*

51 This has been a controversial topic for decades. Wendy Moore in (2005), *The Knife Man: The Extraordinary Life and Times of John Hunter, Father of Modern Surgery*, New York: Broadway Books, summarises quite brilliantly the evidence for her conclusion that Hunter definitely experimented on himself. See endnote 2, pp. 306–7.

52 Hunter, *A Treatise on the Venereal Disease*, p. 326.

John Hunter saved specimens from his patients to show students, 'This is the foot of a patient I had in St. George's Hospital: you see from the sole of the foot what a considerable quantity of this dark fungus arises.' The patient survived.[53]

Hunter instructed his students on how to deal with difficult patients who were in great danger:

> Phymosis and Paraphymosis March 11th 1778
>
> I have seen the complaint so bad as to stop the circulation of the blood beyond the stricture and cause mortification, We often see this complaint in little Boys playing tricks wth. themselves & when I am called to such I never stay the operation of Fermentations etc. for no time can be spared. I take the Penis in my hand & force the Gland back & draw The skin over, never minding his screaming etc. for rough treatment here is necessary – [54]

Maybe it is descriptions like these that led a young William Blake to choose the moniker 'Jack Hunter Tearguts' for *An Island in the Moon*, a piece meant to delight his friends in private. 'Quid the Cynic' (William Blake), 'Suction the Epicurean' (a younger brother) and 'Sipsop the Pythagorean' (William Henry Mathew) host meetings in their homes to discuss the arts and sciences of the day. Mathew was only 15 years old in 1784 and a favourite pupil of John Hunter. Sipsop-Mathew speaks from personal experience of his teacher:

> I only wish Jack *Hunter* Tearguts had had the cutting of Plutarch he understands anatomy better than any of the Ancients hell plunge his knife up to the hilt in a single drive and thrust his fist in. and all in the space of a Quarter of an hour. he does not mind their crying – tho they cry ever so he'll Swear at them & keep then down with his fist & tell that that hell scrape their bones it they don't lay still & be quiet – What. the devil should the people in the hospital that have it done for nothing, make such a piece of work for ...[55]

In fact John Hunter was a great observer of pain:

> No. 26 Amputation of the Leg
> I cut off the leg of a Young Man at St. George's Hospital. A Cart-wheel had passed over his foot, years before, which had disabled him from walking for some time. Under the Operation he behaved extremely well, but from the Wasting of the Limb, and the appearance of the parts, I suspected that the real pain was not so great as is common in such operations.
>
> No. 77 Compound Fracture
> September 1780. A Man came into St. George's Hospital with a very bad compound Fracture. I saw him, not above an hour after he had received the Accident. It appeared to me that the mischief was such as required that the leg should be amputated immediately; and when I proposed it to him, it did not seem to affect him much; from which, and other

53 *Hunterian Reminiscences, Being the Substance of A Course of Lectures on the Principles and Practice of Surgery, delivered by the late Mr John Hunter in the Year 1785*, p. 162. The condition leads to a painful and ultimately fatal, permanent penile erection.

54 Ashmead, f. 279v.

55 Blake, William, *An Island in the Moon*, pp. 39–40.

> Circumstances, I suspected he was drunk, but was told by his friends that he was not. I then began to suspect some other injury, and therefore did not amputate that day.[56]

The patient died the next day and Hunter discovered that a cart wheel had run over his stomach. Pain was a useful diagnostic tool and Hunter not only urged his students to use it but gave numerous instances where it had worked for him:

> On Hydrocele continued
> Where the site of the testicle cannot be determined by the Surgeon, let him have recourse to the feelings of pain. Squeezing the testicle give a different sensation from that arising from squeezing a watery tumour.[57]

As with his predecessors, kitchen nomenclature scatters Hunter's cases – diseased testicles feel like bruised oranges or half-boiled bacon.[58] He tried giving patients a placebo:

> Upon this idea of every gonorrhoea curing itself, I gave certain patients pills of bread which were taken with great regularity. The patients always got well, but some of them I believe not so soon as they would have done had the artificial methods of cure been employed.[59]

The extant cases show that John Hunter dissected at the hospital and at home. He looked for the cause of death and also for any specimens to add to his collection. He also dissected lean subjects to gain knowledge and specimens of their muscles and bones. Lunatics at the lunatic hospital were opened as were bodies brought in from the workhouse. Hunter constantly records how soon after death he opens bodies in terms of hours. Throughout he maintains a calm and dispassionate voice, one that he attempted to instil in his students. Hunter left instructions for his own autopsy and was in fact dissected the day after his death by Everard Home with Matthew Baillie observing and William Clift assisting. Hunter's pupils quietly watched. Contrary to his wishes Hunter's heart and Achilles tendon were not preserved.[60]

The Hunters' legacy

On 7 May 1798 William Clift attended a lecture on 'opening dead bodies' at the Great Windmill Street Anatomy School. The lecturer was James Wilson. In the midst

56 (1993), *The Case Books of John Hunter FRS*, (eds) Allen, Elizabeth, Turk, J.L. and Murley, Sir Reginald, New York: The Parthenon Publishing Group Inc., p. 51. The cases are based on the Transcript of Hunterian Manuscripts contained in two Folio Volumes sent by Sir Everard Home to the Board of Trustees of the Hunterian Collection in 1824 and 1825. Home burnt most of John Hunter's papers in 1800 supposedly to protect his reputation, as Hunter had 'heretical' views. In fact it was to cover up Home's plagiarism of Hunter.

57 Stone, f. 148r.

58 *The Case Books of John Hunter FRS*, p. 61.

59 Ibid., p. 69.

60 Moore, p. 270

of a dry description on how to cut open and examine various organs, Wilson gave this advice on conduct during an autopsy:

> Of great utility to the practitioner himself; also sometimes necessary to satisfy relations. The manner in which a request is made is a great deal towards getting leave. No fee sh.d be required. No parade of instruments, but such as can be put in the one's pocket. Nor go more than one or two to do it. Should have the body out of the coffin if possible – be provided with a pail or two, a jug if you expect fluid to measure it, towels sponges etc. No domestic or relation present if can help it that the surgeons may converse freely or take any part there. Keep the windows so shut as to prevent the neighbours from seeing. If any person is present which prevents you from taking any part you wish, you must endeavour to send them out of the room for something.[61]

Having discussed how to gain access to a body successfully and make preparations to secretly take any interesting bits, Wilson continued with instructions on how to cut open the body and disguise the theft:

> To examine the Thorax & Abdomen make an incision ... . If it be the contents of the bladder ... it may be necessary to make a section of the pubis, must not divide the integuments as the nurses be always are sure to look to these parts afterwards to see that the Doctor has not ran away with them. If the cavities have water in them or you have taken any part out, should fill up again with Bran or Sawdust to prevent from them from thinking you have taken away any part. Should always be very dainty and prevent any appearance of indecency; and then very respectfully inform the friends of the appearances devoid of technical terms as mch. as possible. If you do not find any appearance which is satisfactory to yourself it will be necessary to Humbug the relatives without altogether deviating from truth. Whatever you may discover to have been erroneous in the practice of the first attending practitioner should never be explained to relatives as it can now do no service but only to the practitioner himself.[62]

What are we to make of this passage and its explicit instructions on how to lie, cheat and steal during autopsies? The advice is very similar to that given by William Hunter on how to gain access and how to behave in patients' drawing rooms. Getting a sight of something is what counted to the medical man.

William Hunter's protégés literally clubbed together to fix the prices paid to resurrectionists at a low level. Around 1810 the 'Anatomical Society' included among

---

61 Clift, William, *Lecture One of the Course of Lectures on Anatomy delivered at the Windmill Street School January–May 26th.1798, Lectures by William Cruikshank and Matthew Baillie,* 1798, Royal College of Surgeons, MSS 129, Folder 3, ff.252–4. The quotation is from a lecture found in the back of the manuscript given by James Wilson who was one of the anatomy demonstrators at the school. At the age of 17 William Clift was engaged by John Hunter as his amanuensis and assistant in his museum in 1792. Although he only worked with Hunter for 20 months, Clift spent the rest of his life caring for Hunter's collections and eventually became the first Conservator of the Hunterian Museum. He described John Hunter, in letters home to his family in Cornwall, as 'verry curious', plain in clothes and wigless. Austin, Frances (1991), *The Clift Family Correspondence, 1792–1846*, Sheffield: University of Sheffield, p. 30.

62 Clift, *Lecture One*, f. 254.

others: Everard Home, James Wilson, Matthew Baillie, Astley Cooper, William Clift, and Charles Bell.[63] Bell, a former anatomy instructor of Hunter, purchased a house on Leicester Square for use as an anatomy school. It appears to have soon gained a reputation for being haunted by Mary, 'The Invisible Girl'.[64] She was allegedly a beautiful young woman who was engaged to be married when she died. Several ballads and plays survive concerning Mary's fate. As the poem by Thomas Hood (1799–1845) relates, she was resurrected from St. Mary-le-Bone cemetery and her parts sold to the most famous anatomy teachers in the capital:[65]

Twas in the middle of the night,
To sleep young William tried,
When Mary's ghost came stealing in,
And stood at his bedside.

O William dear! O William dear!
My rest eternal ceases;
Alas! My everlasting peace
Is broken into pieces.

I thought the last of all my cares
Would end with my last minute;
But though I went to my long home
I didn't stay long in it.

The body-snatchers they have come.
And made a snatch of me:
It's very hard them kind of men
Won't let a body be.

You thought that I was buried deep
Quite decent like and chary,
But from her grave in Mary-Bone
They've come and bon'd your Mary.

The arm that used to take your arm
Is took to Dr. Vyse;
And both my legs are gone to walk
The Hospital at Guy's.

63 Richardson, p. 103 and endnotes, pp. 329–30.

64 Shultz, Suzanne M. (1992), *Body Snatching: The Robbing of Graves for the Education of Physicians*, London: McFarland and Co., p. 98.Foot disliked John Hunter as his biography makes clear.

65 St-Mary-le-Bone Cemetery was one of the largest pauper burial grounds in the capital.

I vow'd that you should have my hand,
But fate gives us denial;
You'll find it there, at Dr. Bell's,
In spirits and a phial.

As for my feet, the little feet
You used to call so pretty,
There's one, I know, in Bedford Row,
The t'other's in the city.

I can't tell where my head is gone,
But Doctor Carpue can:
As for my trunk, it's all pack'd up
To go by Pickford's van.

I wish you'd go to Mr. P.
And save me such a ride;
I don't half like the outside place,
They've took for my inside.

The cock it crows – must be gone!
My William, we must part!
But I'll be yours in death, altho'
Sir Astley has my heart.

Don't go to weep upon my grave,
And think that there I be;
They haven't left an atom there
Of my anatomie.[66]

There is some evidence that 'an invisible girl' was actually exhibited at Bell's anatomy school in the early nineteenth century. At least an article titled 'London Teachers of Anatomy: A Retrospect' in the *Lancet* suggests so:

> Charles Bell tk a large ruinous house in Leicester-square, previously inhabited by Speaker Onslow. 'When I got into the house, the first night I slept in it, I had put out the candle, and leaping into bed, the floor gave way under my foot, and I found that I had displaced

66 (*c.*1870), *The Choice Works of Thomas Hood*, New York: Lovell, Wesson, Adam and Company, pp. 191–3. The ballad was published in 1826. A shorter and slightly different version of this poem appears in Graham, Harvey (1943), *The Story of Surgery*, New York: Halcyon House, p. 19. Thomas Hood also composed 'Jack Hall' the story of a bodysnatcher that may be modelled on John Hunter. See Richardson, pp. 173–4. Carpue had an anatomy school in Dean Street and Sir Astley Cooper was a surgeon at Guy's and St Thomas' Hospitals. Bell, Carpue and Astley (Cooper) are listed as receivers of bodies from the Crouch gang in *The Diary of A Resurrectionist 1811–12*. I have not been able to find an anatomist called Dr Vyse.

> the board. On examining this in the morning I discovered a tube under the loose board; it was the house where the "invisible girl" exhibited!'[67]

Thomas Hood was an engraver and a contributor to the *London Magazine.* He had obvious knowledge of the activities and locations of anatomists and their schools. The most famous anatomist he mentioned was the highly successful Sir Astley Cooper, He had attended John Hunter's lectures on anatomy and surgery.[68] In a biography of Astley Cooper, Bransby Blake Cooper depicts his uncle as an educated, rational and sympathetic individual with a certain dispassion due to his love of science – as a pupil of John this would make sense:

> Prejudices such as disgust or fear at the sight of the dead, he could not comprehend, much less tolerate; but for feelings of pain at the idea of mutilation, caused by the affectionate regard of friends and relations to the deceased person, he always felt sympathy. But he would point out, when reasoning on this matter, how soon the grave must produce the same result, and how necessary it was to control feelings which, while they exerted no influence on the dead, were seriously affecting the living: and moreover it would not fail to impress on the educated how necessary it was to set a proper example to those prejudices were increased by ignorance, and who, if they observed the same feelings entertained by their superiors, would not want a justification for any instances to professional inquiries. 'You cannot suppose,' he would conclude by saying, 'that there can be any other gratification in such investigations, than the legitimate one arising from the opportunity it offers, of acquiring fresh knowledge in my profession, and the request which I am urging of you in the cause of science.'[69]

This recollection of Sir Astley Cooper's attitudes towards patients' families and performing autopsies can be compared with an account given by Hampton Weekes (1780–1855) in a letter to his father in 1802. Weekes was an apothecary pupil to Richard Whitfield at St Thomas' Hospital from 1801 to 1803. He became a member of the College of Surgeons in 1802, practised in Brighton and qualified as a physician at the University of Aberdeen in 1808:

> I was present to day when Mr. Cooper examined her body with young Cline and 4 or 5 more, Mr. C. did it in a clandestine manner for her friends had objectd to its being done, – I percieve that you have not been acquainted that she was dead ... ." [a woman of 43 with a ruptured hernia]

---

67 (27 September 1884), *The Lancet*, pp. 535–6. The piece was by Charles Hawkins F.R.C.S.. I have not been able to discover more about this claim to date.

68 Richardson discusses Sir Astley and Bransby Cooper particularly in relation to body snatching and the Anatomy Act of 1832. My interest is more in Astley Cooper's demeanor as surgeon and anatomist and its influence on students.

69 *The Life of Sir Astley Cooper*, Vol.1, p. 105. Astley Cooper tried to keep Resurrectionists out of gaol and if unsuccessful, financially supported their families. Every Christmas he sent a large hamper to Joseph Swan, a surgeon at Lincoln County Hospital. Labelled 'glass with care' it actually contained an adult body for dissection purposes. I thank Mr Oscar Stewart, a former surgeon at the Hospital and now the Director of the Medical Museum, for telling me about this.

> At 4 oClock Mr. Cooper came up into ye. little dissecting room, and dispatched someone after her pretty soon, He laughed with us and said that Mr. Polhill, a great Tobaconist at St. Margaret's Hill, (with Whom this woman had been living), had sent word that she shd. not be inspected, (Mr. P. is also a governor of this Hospital) But ye. answer sh. be to him that she had been open'd before his message had arrived, but wh. was not ye. case, (This shd. not be told to your country Neddy's, neither to any one.) So we were very merry about it, – He took out both Hernia's part of ye. Pubis & Ilium's ...[70]

As with the young James Williams, Weekes's letter reveals his excitement at being in such a clandestine situation. Letters also reveal his struggle to achieve dispassion and that his training in the dissecting room had not totally prepared him for the reality of live surgery. He received this one from his brother:

> Dick desires an explanation of the word tenderness in your Letter, he has a strong inclination to think it is only another name for Sickness, fainting &c &c Dick desires you would remember Elliott, and hopes you was not carried out for a dead man, wishes you to take a bumper of brandy next time & buy you a small bottle of Volatile Salts or a little snuff in a box, but the better way is to take your Eye off at times ...[71]

Seventeen days later, Hampton Weekes was ready to boast of his detachment to Dick, his older brother and a qualified surgeon, but one catches whiffs of his fear and the importance of his peer group in bolstering his dispassion:

> – Mr. Cline operates to morrow on a patient in ye. Hospital for Popliteal aneurism ye. only one since I have been here, at both Hospitalls I have seen operations since I wrote last & mind nothing about it, the more the poor devills cry ye. more I laugh with ye. rest of them, two amputation's of ye. leg one after the other by Chandler (he is in a hurry) a schirrus breast that had ulcerated in a woman, operation for a Hydrocele both by Cooper (a neat operator) they inject red Wine diluted always after tapping it with Trocar ...[72]

There was joy in becoming hardened – new pleasures resulted. Hampton Weekes learned to 'laugh with the rest' and so proclaim mastery of his own body and future mastery of his patients' bodies.

William Hunter and John Hunter shaped young men into medical men in very particular fashions. Through repeated dissections, the Hunters informed their students' heads and gave dexterity to their hands and so linked an intellectual penetration of the body to an instrumental penetration. This familiarized their students' hearts to a sort of 'necessary inhumanity' when it came to treating patients, performing autopsies or

70 Ford, John M.T. (1987), *A Medical Student at St Thomas's Hospital, 1801–2: The Weekes Family Letters*, Medical History, Supplement No.7, London: Wellcome Institute for the History of Medicine, pp. 129–130. The letter is dated 17 February 1802. Henry Cline the elder (1750–1827) attended lectures at both the Hunters' schools and became surgeon to St Thomas'. His son Henry 'young Cline' (1781–1820) became dresser (surgeon's registrar) to his father in 1800, then lecturer in surgery and anatomy in 1811 and surgeon to St Thomas' in 1812.

71 Ford, p. 42. Letter from Richard Weekes, 21 September 1801 to Hampton Weekes.

72 Ibid., p. 49. Letter from Hampton Weekes to Richard Weekes, 8 October 1801. For another account of Cooper operating, see Christison, pp. 197–8.

stealing body parts. Through anatomical therapy the Hunters's protégés became an extension of their teachers. In turn their pupils would become extensions of them. In the process they lost the ability to speak to outsiders but gained a professional identity. William Hunter's lectures and John Hunter's schooling in the dissecting room gave them both a sensory cartography of the body and a common language to communicate their findings to others in the profession. Anatomy did not just fully educate all the senses of young medical men; it was also a gift of moral forbearance. The advice students received on proper conduct around patients and their families was exactly the same as they received on how to handle cadavers in anatomy lessons. Part of the Hunters' legacy was that throughout most of the nineteenth century both spaces – the patient's bedchamber and the operating theatre – came to be regarded as dissecting rooms for members only; members who had been taught to control their feelings and conceal the fact that their cultural attitudes toward death and dismemberment of the body differed radically from that of patients, relatives, neighbours and servants. They were now 'principally conversant with the dead'.

Epilogue

Given the elusive nature of the topic, writing about emotions in history is difficult. I hope that the presentation of a series of case studies of William Harvey, Walter Charleton, John Ward, Daniel Turner, William Hunter and John Hunter has shown that the boundaries and rules of how to behave and what to feel vary not only in time but also in medical culture. The focus of this book has been seventeenth- and eighteenth-century England and how dispassion was taught, debated, learnt and promoted, to whom and why.

My interest in dispassion initially came from many years spent working in health care, as a psychiatric social worker in Britain and as a respiratory therapist and a trauma nurse in America. In all these jobs the question of what to do with your emotions while treating clients and patients loomed large. How should one behave when faced with pain, suffering and death? In the midst of a medical emergency what should one feel or be seen to feel? Objectivity was necessary to render a professional judgement but did objectivity preclude having sympathy for the suffering patient? There was precious little formal training available. Instead learning how to manage emotions was largely absorbed through observing other more seasoned personnel. Junior staff were confusingly told by senior staff that on the one hand they would have to learn detachment, but on the other hand this was a natural process and required no learning. To begin with it was a struggle to practise the rituals and strategies for maintaining calm in the chaotic and violent world of trauma medicine; but, in time and with practice, it developed.'[1] Detached but benevolent professionalism was the goal, with the idea that this protected both the patient and the health-care worker from emotions that would interfere with saving lives. Outside of the profession such detachment could provoke and has provoked condemnation rather than praise.

James Moore, an army surgeon and former pupil of John Hunter, denounced the 'absurd opinion entertained by some people, that a certain degree of cruelty is requisite to enable a man to perform surgical operations with coolness and presence of mind' in *A Method of Preventing or Diminishing Pain in several Operations of Surgery* (1784).[2] Moore soothingly added that:

> ... happily for mankind, the habit of seeing objects of distress, without diminishing the sentiments of compassion in the breasts of the humane, enables them to preserve that

---

1 As Ludmilla Jordanova rightly states, 'medical practice is visual at its heart'. To understand it we 'must study how looking shapes virtually all aspects of medicine', *Locating Medical History*, pp. 354–7. Analysing the architecture of hospitals, the material culture of operating theatres or the clothing chosen for patients and health care workers would reveal much about the desire to create a certain emotional community.

2 Moore, James (1784), *A Method of Preventing or Diminishing Pain in several Operations of Surgery*, London, p. 5. Moore was a surgeon to St George's Hospital in London and was promoting a new method of amputation.

> composure and presence of mind, which is often necessary for giving effectual relief; and which, those to whom distressed objects are less familiar, are exceedingly apt to lose.[3]

Losing pity and gaining control went hand in hand. Hardening or dampening emotions led to heightened perception, knowledge, rationality and a new sensibility – dispassion. It was a hard road to travel as many medical men in this book, and artists such as Leonardo da Vinci, have pointed out:

> I have dissected more than ten human corpses, digging deep into each limb, pulling back the minutest bits of flesh ... If this subject excites you, you may feel a natural repulsion, or even if you're not put off, you may still dread spending the night among cut-up, flayed, ghastly-looking cadavers. If all that still doesn't deter you, you may lack the artistic talent indispensable for this science.[4]

Surely such activities and feelings came at a price – how does medicine shape the man and man the medicine? This is a question that occupied D.J. Weatherall at the beginning of this book and it continues to occupy those within and without the culture of medicine. In 1994 the forensic pathologist Professor Bernard Knight was interviewed by the renowned psychiatrist, Dr Anthony Clare. Knight had performed nearly 30,000 autopsies in his career including ones on genocide victims in Bosnia:

> In this case [Clare] was deeply interested in the character of a man who could stay so calm, apparently unaffected by worse sights than most of us would care to imagine, without even the comfort of religion [malarkey according to Knight]. It transpired that the horror finds its outlet in a recurring dream – also experienced by other pathologists – in which he is performing a post-mortem on a living member of his own family.[5]

It was somehow reassuring to discover that Knight had suffered for learning medical dispassion.

---

3 Ibid., p. 5.

4 Leonardo da Vinci, The Notebooks, *c.*1510, quoted in Comar, Philippe (1999), *Images of the Body,* New York: Harry N. Abrams, Inc., p. 65.

5 Gaisford, Sue (14 August 1994), *Independent*, London, p. 8. This was a review of the Radio Four broadcast.

Bibliography

College of Physicians of Philadelphia

Anonymous (1761), *Dr. David, 2 lectures on dissection*, uncatalogued.
Anonymous (*c.*1783), *Notes taken from Dr. William Hunter's Lectures*, MS 10a/63.
Cline, Henry (*c.*1790), *Lecture on Surgery,* 2/0179–01.
Macgill, James (1753), *A Collection of Manuscripts*, 2/0315–01.

The Folger Shakespeare Library

Ward, John, *Diaries*, V.a. 284–99.
Blome, Grace Randolph (1697), *Her Booke*, V.b. 301.
Power, Sir D'Arcy (1913–26), *Transcript of John Ward's Diaries, 1913–26*, The Folger Shakespeare Library.

The National Library of Medicine

Redman, John (1746), *A Course of Publick Lectures in Anatomy By Alexander Monro, Professor of Anatomy, in the Colledge of Edinburgh,* MS 68–76 no 2.

New York Academy of Medicine

Ashmead, William (28 October 1777), *Physiological Lectures by John Hunter, F.R.S.,* London, MS 10a 165.
Beekman, Fenwick, *Collection of Hunteriana.*
Hunter, John (*c.*1790), *Lectures on Surgery* taken by Richard Stone, London.
Hunter, William (1775), *Anatomical Lectures*, London.

Royal College of Surgeons

Anonymous (1770), *Notes of lectures by William Hunter*, MS 42.c.
Ash, John and Home, Everard (1789), *The Account of the dissection of the Honourable Mr. Howard*, Box 3, Letter 4.
Clift, William (1798), *Lecture One of the Course of Lectures on Anatomy delivered at the Windmill Street School January–May 26th. 1798,* MS 129, Folder 3.
The Diary of A Resurrectionist, MS. 67/a.5.

St Thomas' Hospital, London

Gardiner (1774), *Anatomical Lectures delivered by Sir Joseph Else, Surgeon from October 1774 – April 1775 at his new anatomical Theatre in St. Thomas Hospital.*

Anonymous (*c.*1780), *Introductory Lecture of Mr. William Hunter*, MS 55.

Wellcome Library

Anonymous (1798), *Introductory Lect. Mr Cruikshank 2nd Course Saturday Jan.y 20th 1798*, MS 131.

Anonymous *(c.*1770*)*, *London Medical Student Notebook*, MS 6922.

Mitchell, Patrick (1697–98), *Lecture Notes taken in Paris mainly from the Lectures of Joseph Guichard Duverney at the Jardin du Roi from 1697–8*, London Medical Society, MS 6.

Anonymous (1758), *John Hunters Lectures*, WMS/MSL40 a&b.

Primary Sources:

Adams, Joseph (1801), *Observations on the Cancerous Breast*, London.

Anno secundo & tertio Gulielmi IV. Regis. Cap. LXXV. An Act for regulating Schools of Anatomy, 1st August 1832, section XVI.

Anonymous (1683), *Gideon's Fleece, or The Sieur de Frisk, an heroick Poem. Written on the cursory perusal of a late Book call'd The Conclave of Physicians by a Friend to the Muses*, London.

Anonymous (1715), *An Essay Upon the Duty of Physicians and Patients: The Dignity of Medicine and the Prudentials of Practice, in Two Dialogues,* London.

Anonymous (1740), *A Short Comparative View of the Practice of Surgery in the French Hospitals,* London.

Anonymous (1825), *An Account of the Circumstances Attending the Imprisonment and Death of the late William Millard, London, printed and pub. by Ann Millard*, London.

Baldinger, Ernst Gottfried (1788), *Medicinisches Journal*, Göttingen.

Banister, John (1578), *The Historie of Man, Sucked from the Sappe of the Most Approved Anathomistes, in this Present Age*, London.

Beckett, William (1740), *Practical surgery illustrated and improved: being chirurgical observations with remarks, upon the most extraordinary cases, cures, and dissections, made at St. Thomas's Hospital, Southwark*, London.

Biggs, Noah (1651)*, Mataeotechnia medicinae*: *The vanity of the craft of physick; or, A new dispensatory ...,* London.

Browne, John (1690), *Myographia Nova,* London.

Bullein, William (1562), *Bullein's Bulwarke of Defence Againste all Sicknes, Sornes, and Woundes*, London.

Burnet, Gilbert (1692), *The Bishop of Sarum's Sermon, At the Funeral of the Honourable Robert Boyle, at St. Martins in the Fields, January 7.1691/2*, London.

Cartes, R. des (1650), *The Passions of the Soule,* London.

Castle, George (1667), *The Chymical Galenist*, London.

Cavendish, Margaret (1663), *The Philosophical and Physical Opinions*, London.

Charleton, Walter (1654), *Physiologia, Epicuro-Gassendo-Charltonia: Or a Fabrick of Science Natural upon the Hypothesis of Atoms*.

____. (1656), *Epicurus' Morals*, London.

____. (1657), *The Immortality of the Human Soul*, London.

____. (1659), *Oeconomia animalis*, London.

____. (1664), *A Brief Discourse Concerning the Different Wits of Men*, London.

____. (1668), *The Ephesian and Cimmerian Matrons: two notable examples of the power of love and wit, in the Savoy*, London.

____. (1669), *The Mysterie of Vintners: Or A Brief Discourse concerning the various Sicknesses of WINES, and their respective Remedies, at this Day commonly used*, London.

____. (1674), *Natural History of the Passions*, London.

____. (1680), *Enquiries Into Human Nature in IV Anatomic Praelections in the new Theatre of the Royal Colledge of Physicians in London*, London.

Cheselden, William (1772), *The Anatomy of the Humane Body*, London.

Christison, Robert (1885), *The Life of Robert Christison,* edited by his sons, London.

Clare, P. (1779), *An Essay on the Cure of Abscesses by Caustic*, London.

Clowes, William (1585), *De Morbo Gallico,* London.

____. (1596), *Profitable and necessarie Booke of Medical Observations*, London.

Cooke, James (1685), *Mellificium Chirurgiae: Or, The Marrow of Chirurgery. An Anatomical Treatise*, London.

Cowper, William (1698), *The Anatomy of the Human Body*, London.

De Beer, E.S. (1959), *The Diary of John Evelyn, Kalendarium*, Oxford: Clarendon Press.

Dionis, Pierre (1710), *Course of Chirurgical Operations, Demonstrated in the Royal Gardens at Paris by M. Dionis*, London.

Ent, George (1641), *Apologia pro circulatione sanguinis*, London.

Gale, Thomas (1596), *An Institution of a Chirurgian conteyning the sure Groundes and Principles of Chirurgiry moste necessary and mete for those that will attayne the arte perfectly*, London.

____. (1563), *The Enchiridion, or Manual of Surgery*, London.

____. (1563), *An Excellent treatise on Gunshot Wounds, and the Office of a Surgeon,* London.

Glisson, Francis (1650), *De rachitide,* London.

____. (1654), *Anatomia hepatis,* London.

Gooch, Benjamin (1767), *A Practical Treatise on Wounds and other Chirurgical Subjects to which is Prefixed a Short Historical Account of the Rise and Progress of Surgery and Anatomy*, Norwich.

Goodall, Charles (1676), *The College of Physicians Vindicated, and the True State of Physick in this Nation Faithfully Represented*, London.

____. (1684), *Historical Account of the College's Proceedings Against Empiricks*, London.

____. (1684), *The Royal College of Physicians of London Founded and Established by Law*, London.

Gregory, John (1770), *Observations on the Duties of a Physician*, Manchester.

Grieve, James (1756), *A. Cornelius Celsus of Medicine In Eight Books*, London.

Halle, John (1565), *An Historiall Expostulation: Against the beastlye Abusers, both of Chyrurgerie and Physyke in oure tyme*, London.

Harvey, Gideon (1683), *The Conclave of Physicians, Detecting their Intrigues, Frauds, and Plots, Against their Patients,* London.

Harvey, William (1653), *The Anatomical Exercises of Dr. William Harvey with the Preface of Zachariah Wood Physician of Roterdam,* London.

____. (1653), *Anatomical Exercitations Concerning the Generation of Living Creatures, to which are added particular Discourses, of Births, and of Conceptions, etc.*, London.

____. (1669), *Anatomia Thomae Parri*, in Joannes Betts, *De ortu et natura*, London.

Heister, Lorenz (1745), *A General System of Surgery*, London.

Highmore, Nathaniel (1651), *Corporis humani disquisitio anatomica*, London.

Hood, Thomas (*c.*1870), *The Choice Works of Thomas Hood*, New York: Lovell, Wesson, Adam and Company.

Hooke, Robert (1665), *Micrographia*, London.

Hunter, John (1771), *Natural History of the Human Teeth*, London.

____. (1786), *A Treatise on Venereal Disease,* London.

____. (1786), *Observations on Certain Parts of the Animal Oeconomy*, London.

____. (1794), *Treatise on the Blood Inflammation and Gunshot Wounds*, London.

____. (1784) *Introductory Lectures Delivered by Mr. William Hunter to his last course of Anatomical Lectures at his Theatre in Windmill Street*, London,.

(1833) *Hunterian Reminiscences, Being the Substance of A Course of Lectures on the Principles and Practice of Surgery, delivered by the late Mr John Hunter in the Year 1785*, ed. Parkinson, J.W.K., London: Sherwood, Gilbert and Pepin.

Jenty, Charles Nicholas (1757), *A Course of Anatomico-Physiological Lectures on the Human Structure and Animal Oeconomy*, London.

Johnson, Samuel (1786), *A Dictionary of the English Language in which the words are deduced from their originals*, 8th ed., London.

Lodge, Thomas (1614), *The Workes of Lucius Annaeus Seneca Newly Inlarged and Corrected by Thomas Lodge, D.M.P, London*, London.

Moore, James (1784), *A Method of Preventing or Diminishing Pain in several Operations of Surgery*, London.

(1681), *Musaeum Regalis Societatis or a catalogue and description of the natural and artificial rarities belonging to the Royal Society*, London.

Muys, Jan (1686), *A rational practice of chyrurgery; or, Chyrurgical observations resolved according to the solid fundamentals of true philosophy ... In five decades*, London.

Pare, Ambrose (1565), *Les Oeuvres*, Paris.

Percival, Thomas (1803), *Medical Ethics; or, A Code of Institutes and Precepts Adapted to the professional Conduct of Physicians and Surgeons*, London.

Plot, Robert (1677), *The Natural History of Oxfordshire*, Oxford.

Porter, Samuel (1715), *An Essay Upon the Duty of Physicians and Patients, The Dignity of Medicine and the Prudentials of Practice, in Two Dialogues,* London.

Read, John (1588), *A most excellent and compendious method of curing woundes in the head*, London.

Reid, Alexander (1634), *A Description of the Body of Man*, London.

Report From The Select Committee on Anatomy, Ordered by the House of Commons to be Printed, 22 July 1828.

Riolan, Jean (1653), 'Animadversiones secundae ad Anatomia Reformatam Thomae Bartholini', in *Opuscula nova anatomica*, Paris.

Rivière, Lazare (1672), *The Practice of Physick, comp and trans, Nicolas Culpeper, Abdiah Cole, and William Rowland*, London.

Rowley, William (1774), *A Letter to Dr. William Hunter ... on the Dangerous Tendency of Medical Vanity, occasioned by the death of the late Lady Holland*, London.

____. (1795), *On the Absolute Necessity of Encouraging, Instead of Preventing or Embarrassing the Study of Anatomy. With a Plan to Prevent Violating the Dormitories of the Defunct. Addressed to the Legislature of Great Britain*, London.

Simmons, Simon Foart (1784), *Two Introductory Lectures, delivered by William Hunter, to his last course of Anatomical Lectures, at his Theatre in Windmill-Street: As they were left corrected for the Press by himself. Printed by order of the Trustees, for J. Johnson*, London.

Sprat, Thomas (1667), *History of the Royal Society*, London.

Sprengell, C.J. (1708), *The Aphorisms of Hippocrates and the Sentences of Celsus*, London.

The Trial of John Donellan, Esq., for the wilful Murder, by poison of Sir Theodosius Edward Allesley Boughton, Bart., at the Assizes at Warwick, on Friday, March 20, 1781.

Turner, Daniel (1695), *Apologia Chyrurgica Or A Vindication of the Noble Art of Surgery*, London.

____. (1714), *De Morbis Cutaneis, a Treatise of Diseases incident to the Skin*, London.

____. (1721), *The Art of Surgery*, London.

____. (1729), *The Art of Surgery,* London.

____. (1730), *The Force of the Mother's Imagination upon her Foetus in Utero*, London.

____. (1732), *Syphilis: A Practical Dissertation on the Venereal Disease, in Two Parts,* London.

____. (1733), *The Ancient Physician's Legacy impartially surveyed*, London.

____. (1735), *The Drop and Pill of Mr. Ward considered*, London.

____. (1736), *Aphrodisiacus, a summary of the Ancient Writers on the Venereal Disease*, London.

____. (1739), *A Discourse Concerning Fevers*, London.

Veslingus, Johannes (1653), *The Anatomy of the Body of the Man, wherein is exactly describes every part therof, in the same manner as it is commonly shewed in Publick Anatomies,* London.

Vicary, Thomas (1586), *The Englishemans Treasure*, London.

Watkins, Richard (1651), *Newes from the Dead. Or a true and Exact Narration of the Miraculous deliverance of Anne Greene*, Oxford.

Wharton, Thomas (1656), *Adenographia*, London.

____. (1659), *Diatribae duae*, London.

____. (1664), *Cerebri anatome: cui accesit nervorum descriptio et usus*, London.

____. (1672), *De Anima Brutorum*, London.

Winslow, James Benignus (1743), *An Anatomical Exposition of the Structure of the Human Body*, London.

Wittie, Robert (1651), *Popular errours or the errours of the people in matter of Physick: London,1651. Translated by Robert Wittie, Doctor in Physick from Latin of James Primrose*, London.

Wood, Anthony (1721), *Athenae Oxonienses*, Oxford.

Yonge, James (1679), *Currus Triumphalis,e Terebintho: or an Account of the many admirable vertues of Oleum Terebinthinae*, London.

____. (1682), *Wounds of the Brain proved Curable*, London.

Secondary Sources

Ackerknecht, Edwin (1967), *Medicine at the Paris Hospital, 1794–1848*, Baltimore: The Johns Hopkins Press.

Adams, Aileen K. (1995), 'I am happy in a Wife: A Study of Mrs John Hunter (1714–1801)', Royal College of Surgeons, pp. 32–7.

Allen, Elizabeth, Turk, J.L. and Murley, Sir Reginald (eds) (2201), *The Case Books of John Hunter FRS*, New York: The Parthenon Publishing Group Inc.

Aubrey, John (1898), *Brief Lives,* ed. Clark, Andrew, Oxford: Clarendon Press.

Aveling, J.H. (ed.) (1875), *Memorials of Harvey*, J.&A. Churchill: London.

Ball, James Moore (1989), *The Body Snatchers: Doctors, Grave Robbers and the Law*, New York: Dorset Press.

Balme, Maurice (2000), *Two Antiquaries: A Selection from the Correspondence of John Aubrey and Anthony Wood*, Durham: Durham Academic Press.

Barbour, Reid (1998), *English Epicures and Stoics: Ancient Legacies in Early Stuart Culture*, Amherst: University of Massachusetts Press.

Barker, Peter (1991), 'Stoic contributions to early modern science', in Osler, Margaret, (ed.) *Atoms, pneuma, and tranquillity*, Cambridge and New York: Cambridge University Press, pp. 135–54.

Bartholin, Thomas (1961), *On the Burning of his Library and On Medical Travel*, 1670, translated and introduced by C.D. O'Malley, Lawrence: University of Kansas Libraries.

Beck, Richard T. (1974), *The Cutting Edge: Early History of the Surgeons of London*, London: Royal College of Surgeons.

Becker, Marvin B. (1988), *Civility and Society in Western Europe*, Bloomington: Indiana University Press.

Beekman, Fenwick (1944), 'William Hunter's Education at Glasgow', *Bulletin of the History of Medicine*, **55** (3), pp. 284–97.

Beloved Son Felix: The Journal of Felix Platter a medical student at Montpellier in the Sixteenth Century (1961), translated and introduced by Sean Jennett, London: Frederick Muller Limited.

Benbow, E.W. (1990), 'Medical students' views of necropsies,' *Journal of Clinical Pathology*, **43**, pp. 969–76.

Benfield, Barker, G. (1992), *The Culture of Sensibility: Sex and Society in Eighteenth Century Britain*, Chicago: University of Chicago Press.

Berti-Bock, Premuda, Vial, Rulliere, (1980) 'Le séjour de William HARVEY à Padoue', *Histoire des Sciences Medicales*, **14**, (1), pp. 317–24.

Biagioli, Mario (1993), *Galileo Courtier: The Practice of Science in the Culture of Absolutism. Science and Its Conceptual Foundations*, Chicago: University of Chicago Press.

Blake, James Bailey (ed.), *The Diary of A Resurrectionist 1811–12*, London, (1896).

Blake, William (1987), *An Island in the Moon, A Facsimile of the Manuscript Introduced, Transcribed and Annotated by Michael Phillips*, Cambridge and New York: Cambridge University Press.

Blandy, John P. and Lumley, John S.P. (eds), *The Royal College of Surgeons of England: 200 Years of History at the Millennium*, London: Blackwell Science Ltd, (2000).

Bordo, Susan R. (1987), *The Flight To Objectivity: Essays On Cartesianism & Culture*, New York: State University of New York Press.

Bosatra, Andrea (1954), 'L'organo dell'udito negli studi di Antonio Molinetti anatomico padovano del '600', *Minerva otorinolaringologica,* **4**, pp. 99–102.

Bray, William (1819), *Memoirs illustrative of the life and writings of John Evelyn*, London.

Brazier, Mary A. (1984), *A History of Neurophysiology in the 17th and 18th Centuries: From Concept to Experiment*, New York: Raven Press.

Brockliss, Laurence and Jones, Colin (1997), *The Medical World of Early Modern France*, Oxford: Clarendon Press.

Brown, Theodore (1981), *The Mechanical Philosophy and the 'Animal Oeconomy'*, New York: Arno Press.

____. (1974), 'From Mechanism to Vitalism in Eighteenth-Century Philosophy', *Journal of the History of Biology*, **7** (2), Fall, pp. 179–216.

Browne, Thomas (1970), *Religio Medici* (1643), Menston, England: A Scolar Press facsimile.

Burke, Joseph and Caldwell, Colin (1968), *Hogarth: The Complete Engravings*, London: Thames and Hudson.

Bylebyl, Jerome (1987), 'The School of Padua: Humanistic Medicine in the Sixteenth Century', in Charles Webster (ed.), *Health, Medicine and Mortality in the Sixteenth Century,* Cambridge: Cambridge University Press, pp. 361–3.

Carleton, Samuel (1973), *Pétrone Démoralisé: 'The Ephesian Matron' of John Ogilby*, Ph.D. thesis, University of Texas at Austin.

Castiglioni, Arturo (1941), 'The Origin and Development of the Anatomical Theater to the End of the Renaissance', *Ciba Symposia*, **3** (2), May, pp. 826–44.

Celsus, Aulus Cornelius (1953), 'De re medicina: Book Seven: The Prooemium', in *Medical Works in Facsimile*, London: Pergamum Press.

Carter, Richard B. (1983), *Descartes' Medical Philosophy: The Organic Solution to the Mind-Body Problem*, Baltimore: Johns Hopkins Press.

Chance, Burton (1942), 'Charles Scarborough, An English Educator and Physician to Three Kings', *Bulletin of the History of Medicine*, **12**, pp. 274–96.

Charleton, Walter (1926), *Epicurus' Morals* (1656), introduction by Frederick Manning, London: Peter Davies.

____. (1975), *The Ephesian Matron* (1668), introduction by Achsah Guibbory, Los Angeles: William Andrews Clark Memorial Library.

Charlton, Roger (1994), 'Autopsy and medical education: a review', *Journal of the Royal Society of Medicine,* **87**, April, pp. 232–6.

Clark, Sir George (1964–66), *A History of the Royal College of Physicians of London*, Oxford: Clarendon Press.

Clericuzio, Antonio (2000), *Elements, Principles and Corpusles: A Study of Atomism and Chemistry in the Seventeenth Century*, Boston: Kluwer Academic Publishers, pp. 92–100.

Cook, Harold J. (1994), *Trials of an Ordinary Doctor: Joannes Groenevelt in Seventeenth-Century London*, Baltimore: Johns Hopkins University Press.

____. (January, 1994), 'Good Advice and Little Medicine', *Journal of British Studies,* **33**, pp. 1–31.

____.(1986), *The Decline of the Old Medical Regime in Stuart London*, Ithaca: Cornell University Press.

Cole, F.J. (1914), *History of the Anatomical Museum*, London.

Comar, Philippe (1999), *Images of the Body,* New York: Harry N. Abrams, Inc.

Copeman, W.S.C. (1960), *Doctors and Disease in Tudor Times*, London: Dawson's of Pall Mall.

Corner, Betsy Copping (1951), 'Dr. Ibis and the Artists: A Sidelight upon Hunter's Atlas, *The Gravid Uterus*', *Journal of the History of Medicine and Allied Sciences*, **1**, pp. 1–21.

Costello, William T. (1958), *The Scholastic Curriculum at Early Seventeenth-Century Cambridge*, Cambridge, Mass.: Harvard University Press.

Cunningham, Andrew (1997), *The Anatomical Renaissance: The Resurrection of the Anatomical Projects of the Ancients*, Cambridge: Cambridge University Press.

____. (1996), 'Sir Thomas Browne and Religio Medici', in Grell, Ole Peter and Cunningham, Andrew (eds), *Religio Medici: Medicine and Religion in Seventeenth-Century England*, Aldershot: Scolar Press, pp. 12–61.

____. (1996), 'The historical context of Wharton's work on the glands', in Freer, Stephen and Cunningham, Andrew, *Thomas Wharton's Adenographia*, Oxford: Clarendon Press, pp. 27–52.

Davis, Audrey (1973), *Circulation Physiology and Medical Chemistry in England 1650–1800*, New York: Coronado Press.

De Beer, E.S. (ed.) (1955), *The Diary of John Evelyn*, Oxford: Clarendon Press.

De Moulin, Daniel (1983), *A Short History of Breast Cancer*, Boston: Martinus Nijhoff Publishers Group.

Dear, Peter (1988), 'A Mechanical Microcosm: Bodily Passions, Good Manners, and Cartesian Mechanism', in Lawrence, Christopher and Shapin, Steven, (eds) *Science Incarnate, Historical Embodiments of Natural Knowledge*, Chicago: University of Chicago Press, pp. 51–82.

Debus, Allen G. (1974), 'Paracelsian Medicine: Noah Biggs and the Problem of Medical Reform', in Debus, Allen G. (ed.), *Medicine in Seventeenth Century England*, Berkeley: University of California Press, pp. 33–48.

Descartes, Rene, (1972), *Treatise of Man*, trans. Thomas Steele Hall, Cambridge, MA: Harvard University Press.

Dewhurst, Kenneth (1980), *Willis' Oxford Lectures*, Oxford: Sandford Publications.

Dingwall, Helen M. (1995), *Physicians, Surgeons and Apothecaries: Medicine in Seventeenth Century Edinburgh*, Edinburgh: Tuckwell Press.

Dobbs, B.J. Teeter and Jacob, Margaret C. (1995), *Newton and the Culture of Newtoniasm*, New Jersey: Humanities Press.

Dobbs, B.J. Teeter (1991), *The Janus Face of Genius: The Role of Alchemy in Newton's Thought*, Cambridge: Cambridge University Press.

Dobson, Jesse and Walker, R. Milnes (1979), *Barbers and Barber-Surgeons of London*, Oxford: Alden Press.

Dobson, Jesse (1969), *John Hunter*, Edinburgh: E. & S. Livingstone Ltd.

____. (1953), 'Observables at the Royal College of Surgeons. 42 Charles Byrne: The Irish Giant', *Annals of the Royal College of Surgeons of England*, **13** (1), July, pp. 63–5.

Douglas, Aileen (1995), *Uneasy Sensations: Smollett and the Body*, Chicago: University of Chicago Press.

Duden, Barbara (1991), *The Woman Beneath the Skin. A Doctor's Patients in Eighteenth Century Germany*, trans. Thomas Dunlap, Cambridge, MA: Harvard University Press.

Durey, M.J. (1976), 'Body snatchers and Benthamites: The Implications of the Dead Body Bill for the London Schools of Anatomy, 1820–42', *The London Journal*, **2** (2), pp. 200–25.

Edwards, G. (1968), 'John Hunter's Last Pupil,' *Annals of the Royal College of Surgeons of England*, **42**, pp. 68–70.

Elias, Norbert (1971), *The Civilizing Process*: *The Development of Manners*, trans. E. Jephcott, New York: Pantheon.

Ellis, Harold (1969), *A History of the Bladder Stone*, Oxford: Blackwell Scientific Publications.

Erickson, Robert A. (1993), 'William Harvey's *De motu cordis* and The Republick of Literature', *Literature and Medicine During the Eighteenth Century*, Roberts, Marie Mulvey and Porter, Roy (eds), London: Routledge, pp. 58–83.

Eriksson, R. (ed.) (1959), *Andreas Vesalius' First public anatomy at Bologna 1540. An eyewitness report by Baldasar Heseler, together with his notes on Matthaeus Curtius' Lectures on Anatomia Mundini*, Uppsala: Uppsala University Press.

Evans, Robert C. (1992), *Jonson, Lipsius and The Politics of Renaissance Stoicism*, Wakefield, N.H.: Longwood Academic Press.

Faber, Richard (1983), *The Brave Courtier: Sir William Temple*, London: Faber and Faber.

Ferrari, Giovanna (1987), 'Public Anatomy Lessons and the Carnival in Bologna', *Past and Present*, **117**, November, pp. 50–106.

Findlen, Paula (1994), *Possessing Nature: Museums, Collecting, And Scientific Culture in Early Modern Italy*, Berkeley: University of California Press.

Fissell, Mary (1991), *Patients, Power and the Poor in Eighteenth-Century Bristol*, Cambridge and New York: Cambridge University Press.

Ford, John M.T. (1987), *A Medical Student at St Thomas's Hospital, 1801–2: The Weekes Family Letters*, Medical History, Supplement No.7, Wellcome Institute for the History of Medicine.

Fothergill-Payne, Louise (1991), 'Seneca's role in popularizing Epicurus in the sixteenth century', in Osler, Margaret (ed.), *Atoms, pneuma, and tranquillity*, Cambridge and New York: Cambridge University Press, pp. 115–33.

Foucault, Michel (1973), *The Birth of the Clinic: An Archaeology of Medical Perception*, New York: Vintage Books.

Fox, Renee C. and Lief, Harold I. (1963), 'Training for "Detached concern" in Medical Students', in Lief, Harold I., Lief, Victor F. and Lief, Nina R. (eds), *The Psychological Basis of Medical Practice by 52 Authors*, New York: Hoeber Medical Division, pp. 12–35.

Frank, Jr, Robert G. (1974), 'The John Ward Diaries: Mirror of Seventeenth Century Science and Medicine', *Journal of the History of Medicine*, **49**, pp. 147–79.

____. (1980), *Harvey and the Oxford Physiologists: A Study of Scientific Ideas,* Los Angeles: University of California Press.

____. (1979), 'The Image of Harvey in Commonwealth and Restoration England', in Bylebyl, Jerome J. (ed.), *William Harvey and His Age: The Professional and Social Context of the Discovery of Circulation*, Baltimore: John Hopkins University Press, pp. 103–36.

____. (1994) 'Medicine' in *The History of the University of Oxford*, Vol. IV, Oxford: Oxford University Press, Tyacke, Nicholas (ed.), pp. 505–58.

____. (1979), *English Scientific Virtuosi in the 16th and 17th Centuries*, Los Angeles: William Andrews Clark Library.

Fraser, Antonia (1973), *Cromwell, Our Chief of Men*, London: Weidenfeld and Nicolson.

French, Roger (1989), 'Harvey in Holland: circulation and the Calvinists', in French, Roger and Wear, Andrew (eds), *The Medical Revolution of the Seventeenth Century*, Cambridge and New York: Cambridge University Press, pp. 46–86.

____. (1994), *William Harvey's Natural Philosophy*, Cambridge and New York: Cambridge University Press.

Gaisford, Sue (14 August 1994), *Independent*, London, p. 8.

Gascoigne, John (1990), 'A reappraisal of the role of the universities in the Scientific Revolution', in Lindberg, David C. and Westman, Robert S. (eds), *Reappraisals of the Scientific Revolution*, Cambridge: Cambridge University Press, pp. 207–60.

Gaukroger, Stephen (1995), *Descartes: An Intellectual Biography*, Oxford: Clarendon Press.

Gelbart, Nina Rattner (1971), 'The Intellectual Development of Walter Charleton', *Ambix*, **18** (3), November, pp. 149–68.

Gelfand, Toby (1980), *Professionalizing Modern Medicine: Paris Surgeons and Medical Science and Institutions in the 18th Century*, Westport: Westport CT. Press.

____. (1985), ' "Invite the Philosopher, As Well as the Charitable": Hospital Teaching as Private Enterprise in Hunterian London', in Bynum, William and Porter, Roy (eds), *William Hunter and the Eighteenth Century Medical World*, Cambridge and New York: Cambridge University Press, pp. 129–52.

____. (1981), 'Gestation of the Clinic,' *Medical History,* **25**, pp. 169–80.

____. (1972), 'The "Paris Manner" of Dissection: Student Anatomical Dissection in Early Eighteenth Century Paris', *Bulletin of the History of Medicine*, **46** (2), March–April, pp. 99–130.

____. (1984), 'A "Monarchial Profession" in the Old Regime: Surgeons, Ordinary Practitioners, and Medical Professionalization in Eighteenth-Century France', in Genson, R. (ed.), *Professions and The French State, 1700–1900*, Philadelphia: Pennsylvania State Press.

Geyer-Kordesch, Johanna and MacDonald, Fiona (1999), *The History of the Royal College of Physicians and Surgeons of Glasgow 1599–1858*, London: The Hambledon Press.

Getz, Faye M. (1992), 'The Faculty of Medicine before 1500', in Catto, J.I. and Evans, Ralph (eds), *The History of the University of Oxford*, Oxford: Clarendon Press, **2**, pp. 373–409.

Gloyne, Roodhouse (1950), *John Hunter*, Edinburgh: E. & S. Livingstone Ltd.

Goffman, Erving (1974), 'The Operating Room: A Study in Role Distance', in Wrong, Dennis H. and Gracey, Harry L., (eds), *Readings in Introductory Sociology*, New York: Macmillan Co., pp. 94–103.

Graham, Harvey (1943), *The Story of Surgery*, New York: Halcyon House.

Greenblatt, Stephen (1980), *Renaissance Self-Fashioning from More to Shakespeare*, Chicago: University of Chicago Press.

Griffin, Jr, Martin I.J. (1992), *Latitudinarianism in the Seventeenth Century Church of England*, Leiden: Brill Academic Publishers.

Gittings, Clare (1984), *Death, Burial and the Individual in Early-Modern England*, London: Croom Helm.

Haas, Jack and Shaffir, William (1992), *Becoming Doctors: The Adoption of a Cloak of Competence*, Greenwich, Conn.: Jai Press Inc.

Hafferty, Frederic W. (1991), *Into the Valley: Death and the Socialization of Medical Students,* New Haven: Yale University Press.

Hall, A. Rupert and Hall, Marie Boas (eds) (1996), *The Correspondence of Henry Oldenburg*, Madison: University of Wisconsin Press.

Hall, Thomas S. (1969), *The History of General Physiology*, Chicago: University of Chicago Press.

Harley, David (1993), 'Ethics and Dispute Behaviour in the Career of Henry Bracken of Lancaster: Surgeon, Physician and Man Midwife', in Baker, Robert, Porter,

Dorothy and Porter, Roy (eds), *The Codification of Medical Morality: Historical and Philosophical Studies of the Formalization of Western Medical Morality in the Eighteenth and Nineteenth Centuries*, Dordrecht: Kluwer Academic Publications, pp. 19–45.

____. Harley, David (1994), 'The Good Physician and the Godly Doctor: The Exemplary Life of John Tylston of Chester (1663–99)', *The Seventeenth Century Journal*, **9** (1), Spring, pp. 1–31.

____. (July 1994), 'Political Post-mortems and Morbid Anatomy in Seventeenth-Century England', *Social History of Medicine*, **7** (1), pp. 1–28.

Harris, Frances (2003), *Transformation of Love: The Friendship of John Evelyn and Margaret Godolphin*, Oxford: Oxford University Press.

Harris, Tim, Seaward, Paul and Goldie, Mark (eds) (1990), *The Politics of Religion in Restoration England*, London: Blackwell.

Harth, Erica (1992), *Cartesian Women: Versions and Subversions of Rational Discourse in the Old Regime*, Ithaca: Cornell University Press.

Harvey, William (1963), *On the Motion of the Heart and Blood in Animals*, trans. Thomas Willis, revised and edited by Alexander Bowie, Chicago: Gateway Editions.

Harvey, William (1995), *The Anatomical Exercises: De Motu Cordis and De Circulatione Sanguinis in English Translation*, ed. Keynes, Geoffrey, New York: Dover Publications.

____. (1961), *Lectures on the Whole of Anatomy: An Annotated Translation of Prelectiones Anatomiae Universalis*, O'Malley, C.D., Poynter, F.N.L. and Russell, K.F. (eds), Berkeley: University of California Press.

____. (1981), *Disputations touching the generation of animals*, translated with an introduction and notes by Gweneth Whitteridge, Oxford: Oxford University Press.

Haslam, Fiona (1996), *From Hogarth to Rowlandson: Medicine in Art in Eighteenth-Century Britain*, Liverpool: Liverpool University Press.

Henry, John (1992), 'The Scientific Revolution in England', in Porter, Roy and Teich, Mikuláš (eds), *The Scientific Revolution in National Context*, Cambridge and New York: Cambridge University Press, pp. 178–209.

Herbert, George (1941), *Works*, ed. Hutchinson, F.E., Oxford: Clarendon Press.

Heyd, Michael (1995), '*Be Sober and Reasonable: The Critique of Enthusiasm in the Seventeenth and Early Eighteenth Centuries*, Leiden: E.J. Brill.

Hirschauer, Stefan (1991), 'The Manufacture of Bodies in Surgery', *Social Studies of Science*, **21**, pp. 279–319.

Holger-Maehle, Andreas (1993) 'The Ethical Discourse on Animal Experimentation, 1650–1900', in Wear, Andrew Geyer-Kordesch, Johanna and French, Roger (eds), *Doctors and Ethics: The Earlier Historical Setting of Professional Ethics*, Amsterdam: Rodolphi Press, pp. 203–51.

Hunter, Richard A. and Cuttler, Emily (1958), 'Walter Charleton's Natural History of the Passions (1674) and J.F. Senault's The Use of Passions (1649): A Case of Mistaken Identity', *Journal of the History of Medicine*, January, **33**, pp. 87–92.

Hunter, Michael (1981), *Science and Society in Restoration England*, Cambridge and New York: Cambridge University Press.

Hunter's Lectures of Anatomy (1972), Amsterdam: Elsevier Publishing Company.

(1939), *Index biographique des membres et correspondants de l'academie des sciences de 1666 a 1939,* Paris: Etudes decouverte.

Jacyna, Stephen (1992), 'Physiological principles in the surgical writings of John Hunter', in Lawrence, Christopher, *Medical Theory: Surgical Practice*, London: Routledge, pp. 135–52.

Jensen, H. James (ed.) (1996), *The Sensational Restoration*, Bloomington: Indiana University Press.

Jewson, N.D. (September 1976), 'The Disappearance of the Sick-Man from Medical Cosmology, 1770–1870', *Sociology*, **10** (3), pp. 225–44.

Johns, Adrian (1996), 'The Physiology of Reading and the Anatomy of Enthusiasm', Grell, Ole Peter and Cunningham, Andrew (eds), *Religio Medici: Medicine and Religion in Seventeenth-Century England*, Aldershot: Scolar Press, pp. 136–70.

Jones, Peter Murray (1988), 'Thomas Lorkyn's Dissections, 1564/5 and 1566/7', *Transactions of the Cambridge Bibliographical Society*, **9**, pp. 209–29.

Jordanova, Ludmilla (1985), 'Gender, generation and science: William Hunter's obstetrical atlas', in Bynum, William and Porter, Roy (eds), *William Hunter and the Eighteenth Century Medical World*, Cambridge and New York: Cambridge University Press, pp. 387–412.

Kaplan, Jonathan (2001), *The Dressing Station: A Surgeon's Chronicle of War and Medicine,* London: Grove Press.

Keele, Kenneth D. (1965), *William Harvey: The man, the physician, and the scientist*, London and Edinburgh: Thomas Nelson Printers Ltd.

____. (1962), 'William Harvey as Morbid Anatomist', *Proceedings of the Royal Society*, **55**, August, pp. 677–84.

Keevil, J.J. (1957), *Medicine and the Navy: 1200–1900*, Edinburgh: E. & S. Livingstone Ltd.

Kemp, Martin (1975), *Dr William Hunter at the Royal Academy of Arts*, Glasgow: University of Glasgow Press.

Keynes, Geoffrey (1966), *The Life of William Harvey*, Oxford: Clarendon Press.

Klestinec, Cynthia (2004), 'A History of Anatomy Theaters in Sixteenth-Century Padua', *Journal of the History of Medicine and Allied Sciences*, **59** (3), pp. 375–412.

Knott, John (1985), 'Popular Attitudes to Death and Dissection in Early Nineteenth Century Britain: The Anatomy Act and the Poor', *Labour History* (Canberra), **49**, pp. 1–18.

Komp, Diane M. (September/October 1994), 'Closing the Distance', *Physician*, pp. 11–12.

Kraus, Robert E. (1988), *Walter Charleton and The Natural History of Nutrition: Galenism in the Scientific Revolution*, MA thesis, University of North Carolina, Chapel Hill.

Kroll, Richard W.F. (1991), *The Material Word: Literate Culture in the Restoration and the Early Eighteenth Century*, Baltimore: The Johns Hopkins University Press.

Kuriyama, Shigehisa (1984), 'Pulse Diagnosis in the Greek and Chinese Traditions', in Kawakita, Yosio (ed.), *History of Diagnostics*, Shiznoka, Japan: The Taniguchi Foundation Suosono-shi.

Lane, Joan (1996), *Apprenticeship in England, 1600–1914*, London: University College London Press Limited, pp. 131–3.

____. (1988), 'Provincial Medical Apprentices and Masters in Early Modern England', *Eighteenth Century Life*, **12** (3), pp. 14–27.

Lansdowne, Marquis of (ed.), (1927), *The Petty Papers*, London.

Latham, Robert (ed.), (1985), *The Shorter Pepys*, Berkeley: University of California Press.

Lawrence, Christopher (1988), 'Alexander Monro *Primus* and the Edinburgh Manner of Anatomy', *Bulletin of Medical History*, **62**, pp. 193–214.

Lawrence, Susan C. (1995), 'Anatomy and Address: Creating Medical Gentlemen in Eighteenth-Century London', Nutton, Vivian and Porter, Roy (eds), *The History of Medical Education in Britain*, Amsterdam: Rodolphi Press, pp. 199–228.

____. (1996), *Charitable Knowledge: Hospital pupils and practitioners in eighteenth-century London*, Cambridge: Cambridge University Press.

Le Gallienne, Richard (ed.), (2001), *The Diary of Samuel Pepys*, New York: The Modern Library.

Lindeboom, Dr G.A. (1979), *Descartes and Medicine*, Amsterdam: Rodolphi Press.

Linebaugh, Peter (1975), 'The Tyburn Riot Against the Surgeons', in Douglas Hay et al (eds), *Albion's Fatal Tree: Crime and Society in Eighteenth-Century England*, New York: Pantheon Books, pp. 65–117.

Long, Esmond R. (1929), 'William Harvey to Jean Riolan, 1649', trans. Willis, Robert, *Selected Readings in Pathology*, Baltimore: Thomas Press.

Lunsingh Scheurleer, Th. H. (1975), 'Un Amphithéâtre D'Anatomie Moralisée', in Th. H. Lunsingh Scheurleer and G.H.M. Posthumus Meyjes (eds), *Leiden University in the Seventeenth Century: An Exchange of Learning*, Leiden: Leiden University Press, pp. 217–77.

Macgee, Reginald (2003), 'Writings of Daniel Turner and his views on the practice of surgery', *ANZ. Journal of Surgery*, **73**, pp. 438–42.

Malloch, Archibald (1917), *Finch and Baines: A Seventeenth Century Friendship*, Cambridge: Cambridge University Press.

Mandelbrote, Scott, 'William Petty and Anne Greene: Medical and Political Reform in Commonwealth Oxford', in (2001) Pelling, Margaret and Mandelbrote, Scott (eds), *The Practice of Reform in Health, Medicine, and Science, 1500–2000*, Aldershot and Burlington, VT: Ashgate Press, pp. 125–49.

Mann, Ronald D. (ed.) (1985), *The History of the Management of Pain*, New Jersey: Parthenon Publishing Group.

Marburg, Clara (1932), *Sir William Temple: A Seventeenth Century 'Libertin'*, New Haven: Yale University Press.

Martensen, Robert (1992), '"Habit of Reason": Anatomy and Anglicanism in Restoration England', *Bulletin of the History of Medicine*, **66**, pp. 511–35.

____. (2004), *The Brain Takes Shape: An Early History*, Oxford: Oxford University Press.

____. (1992), 'The Transformation of Eve: Women's Bodies, Medicine and Culture in Early-Modern England', in Porter, Roy (ed.), *Sexual Knowledge. Sexual Science: The History of Attitudes to Sexuality*, Cambridge and New York: Cambridge University Press, pp. 107–33.

McGrath, Roberta (2002), *Seeing Her Sex: Medical Archives and the Female Body*, Manchester: Manchester University Press.

Medvei, Victor Cornelius and Thornton, John L. (1974), *The Royal Hospital of Saint Bartholomew 1123–1973*, London: The Royal Hospital of Saint Bartholomew.

Missen, John and Hill, Dennis, 'The Anatomy Theatre', in Burns, Ian (ed.), *The Company of Barbers and Surgeons*, London: The Worshipful Company of Barbers, pp. 111–28.

Mol, Annemarie (2002), *The Body Multiple: Ontology in Body Practice*, Durham, NC: Duke University Press.

Moore, Wendy (2005), *The Knife Man: The Extraordinary Life and Times of John Hunter, Father of Modern Surgery*, New York: Broadway Books.

Morford, Mark (1991), *Stoics and Neostoics: Rubens and the Circle of Lipsius*, Princeton: Princeton University Press.

Murray, Ian and Hall, Brian (2000), 'The Hall and the area in which we live', in Burns, Ian (ed.), *The Company of Barbers and Surgeons*, London: The Worshipful Company of Barbers, pp. 45–60.

Nicolson, Marjorie Hope (ed.) (1930), *Conway Letters: The Correspondence of Anne, Viscountess Conway, Henry More, and their Friends, 1642–1684*, New Haven: Yale University Press.

Niebyl, Peter H. (1971), '"The Non Naturals": A Note on the Origins and Fate of a Doctrine and a Phrase', *Bulletin of the History of Medicine*, **45**, pp. 486–92.

(The) Note-Book of Edward Jenner (1931), with an introduction by Drewitt, F. Dawtrey, London: Oxford University Press.

Nutton, Vivian (May 1995), '"A diet for barbarians": Introducing Renaissance Medicine to Tudor England', unpublished paper given at the *Dibner Institute Conference on Natural Philosophy and the Disciplines in Early-Modern Europe*.

O'Malley, C.D. (1967), 'John Evelyn and Medicine', *Medical History*, **12**, pp. 219–31.

Oestreich, Gerhard, Oestreich, Brigitta and Koenigsberger, H.G. (eds) (1982), *Neostoicism and the early modern state*, trans. McLintock, David, Cambridge and New York: Cambridge University Press.

Osler, Margaret J. (1979), 'Descartes and Charleton on Nature and God', *Journal of the History of Ideas*, **40** (3), pp. 445–56.

Ottley, Drewry (1835), *The Life of John Hunter*, London.

Pagel, Walter (1967), *William Harvey's Biological Ideas,* New York: Karger.

____. (1976), *New Light on William Harvey*, New York: Karger.

Paget, Stephen (1897), *John Hunter: Man of Science and Surgeon*, London: T. Fisher Unwin.

Park, Katharine (1994), 'The Criminal and Saintly Body: Autopsy and Dissection in Renaissance Italy', **47**, *Renaissance Quarterly*, pp. 1–33.

Paster, Gail Kern, Rowe, Katherine, Floyd-Wilson, Mary (eds) (2004), *Reading the Early Modern Passions: Essays in the Cultural History of Emotion*, Philadelphia: University of Pennsylvania Press.

Payne, Lynda (2002), 'With much nausea, loathing, and foetor: William Harvey, dissection and dispassion in early modern medicine.' *Vesalius: Acta Internationales Historiae Medicinae*, **3** (2), December, pp. 45–52.

Peachey, George (1924), *A Memoir of William and John Hunter*, Plymouth.

Pelling, Margaret (1985), 'Appearance and Reality: barber-surgeons, the body and disease', in Beier, A.L. and Finlay, Roger (eds), *London 1500–1700: The Making of a City*, London: Longmans, pp. 82–112.

Phillips, Salman (1992), 'William Harvey and Art Misplaced', *Annals of Science*, **49**, pp. 3–19.

Porter, Dorothy and Porter, Roy (1989), *Patient's Progress: Doctors and Doctoring in Eighteenth-Century England*, Stanford: Stanford University Press.

Porter, Roy (1987), 'The language of quackery in England, 1660–1800', in Burke, Peter and Porter, Roy (eds), *The Social History of Language*, Cambridge and New York: Cambridge University Press, pp. 73–103.

____. (1989), *Health for Sale: Quackery in England 1660–1850*, Manchester: Manchester University Press.

____. (1995), 'Medical Lecturing in Georgian London', *The British Journal of the History of Science*, **28** (96), March, pp. 91–9.

____. (1995), 'The Eighteenth Century', in Conrad, Neve, Nutton, Porter and Wear (eds), *The Western Medical Tradition: 800 B.C. to A.D. 1800*, Cambridge and New York: Cambridge University Press, pp. 371–476.

____. (2000), *Quacks: Fakers and Charlatans in English Medicine*, London: Tempus.

Power, Sir D'Arcy (1886), *Memorials of the Craft of Surgery in England*, London: Cassell and Co.

____. (1917), *Trans. med. Soc. Lond.* **40**, pp. 1–26.

____. (1920), *Trans. med. Soc. Lond*, **43**, pp. 253–84.

____. (1931), *Selected Writings*, London, pp. 173–200.

Proctor, Judith (1995), *The Suffering Self: Pain and Narrative Representation in the Early Christian Era*, New York and London: Routledge.

Rawcliffe, Carole (1995), *Medicine and Society in Later Mediaeval England*, Stroud, Gloucestershire: Alan Sutton.

Reddy, William M. (2001), *The Navigation of Feeling: A Framework for the History of Emotions*, Cambridge and New York: Cambridge University Press.

Rey, Roselyne (1993), *History of Pain*, trans. Wallace, Louise Elliott, Cadden, J.A., and Cadden, S.W., Paris: Editions la Decouverte.

Richardson, Ruth (2001), *Death, Dissection and the Destitute*, Chicago: University of Chicago Press.

____. (1996), 'Fearful Symmetry: Corpses for Anatomy, Organs for Transplantation?' in Youngner, Stuart J., Fox, Renee C. and O'Connell, Laurence J. (eds), *Organ Transplantation: Meanings and Realities*, Madison: University of Wisconsin Press, pp. 66–100.

Robb-Smith, A.H.T. (1986), 'Medical Education at Oxford and Cambridge prior to 1850', in Poynter, F.N.L. (ed.), *The Evolution of Medical Education in Britain*, Baltimore: The Williams and Wilkins Co.

Rolleston, Humphrey (1940), 'Walter Charleton, D.M., F.R.C.P., F.R.S', *Bulletin of the History of Medicine*, **8**, pp. 403–16.

Rosenwein, Barbara (June 2002), 'Review Essay: Worrying about Emotions in History', *American History Review* **107** (3), pp. 821–45.

Ross, Ian and Ross, Carol Urquhart (1980), 'Body Snatching in Nineteenth Century Britain: From Exhumation to Murder', *British Journal of Law and Society*, **6**, (1), pp. 108–18.

Rousseau, G.S. (1999) "'Stung in to action ...": Medicine Professionalism, and the News', in Raymond, Joad (ed.), *News, Newspapers, and Society in Early Modern Britain*, London: Frank Cass and Company, pp. 176–205.

Rupke, Nicolaas A. (ed.) (1987), *Vivisection in Historical Perspective,* London: Croom Helm.

Rupp, Jan (1990), 'Matters of Life and Death: the social and cultural conditions of the rise of anatomical theaters, with special reference to seventeenth century Holland', *History of Science*, **28**, pp. 264–87.

____. (1992), 'Michel Foucault, Body Politics and the Rise and Expansion of Modern Anatomy', *Journal of Historical Sociology*, **5** (1), March, pp. 31–59.

Saunders, Jason Lewis (1955), *Justus Lipsius: The Philosophy of Renaissance Stoicism*, New York: The Liberal Arts Press.

Sawday, Jonathan (1995), *The Body Emblazoned: Dissection and the Human Body in Renaissance Culture*, London and New York: Routledge.

Scarry, Elaine (1985), *The Body in Pain*, Berkeley: University of California Press.

Schaffer, Simon (1980), 'Natural Philosophy', in Rousseau, G.S. and Porter, Roy, (eds), *The Ferment of Knowledge*, Cambridge: Cambridge University Press, pp. 53–92.

____. (1983), 'Natural Philosophy and Public Spectacle in the Eighteenth Century', *History of Science*, **21**, pp. 1–43.

Schotzinger, Kathleen A. and Best, Elizabeth Kirkley (1987–88), 'Closure and the Cadaver Experience: A Memorial Service for Deeded Bodies', *Omega: Journal of Death and Dying*, **18** (3), pp. 217–227.

Scodel, Joshua (2002), *Excess and the Mean in Early Modern Literature*, Princeton: Princeton University Press.

Severn, Charles (1839), *Diary of Rev. John Ward, A.M.*, London.

Shaaber, M.A. (ed.) (1957), *Seventeenth Century Prose*, New York: Harper & Brothers Publishers.

Shapin, Steven (1990), 'The Mind Is Its Own Place: Science and Solitude in Seventeenth-Century England', *Science in Context*, **4**, (1), pp. 191–218.

____. (1994), *A Social History of Truth: Civility and Science in Seventeenth-Century England*, Chicago: University of Chicago Press.

Shapin, S. and Schaffer, S. (1989), *Leviathan and the Air-Pump*, Princeton: Princeton University Press.

Sharp, Lindsay (1973), 'Walter Charleton's Early Life 1620–1659, and Relationship to Natural Philosophy in Mid-Seventeenth Century England', *Annals of Science*, **30**, pp. 311–40.

Shaw, A. Batty (1972), 'Benjamin Gooch, Eighteenth-Century Norfolk Surgeon', *Medical History*, **16**, pp. 40–50.

Shultz, Suzanne M. (1992), *Body Snatching: The Robbing of Graves for the Education of Physicians*, London: McFarland and Co.

Siena, Kevin (2004), *Venereal Disease, Hospitals and the Urban Poor*, Rochester: University of Rochester Press.

Silverman, Lisa (2001), *Tortured Subjects: Pain, Truth, and the Body in Early Modern France*, Chicago: University of Chicago Press.

Simmons, Simon Foart (1983), *William Hunter, 1718–1783: a memoir*, Brock, C.H. (ed.), Glasgow: Glasgow University Press.

Small, Carole and Small, Alistair (1997), 'John Evelyn and the Garden of Epicurus', *Journal of the Warburg and Courtauld Institutes*, **60**, pp. 194–214.

Sommerville, C. John (1989) *Popular Religion in Restoration England*, Gainesville, Fla.: University Press of Florida.

Spurr, John (1991), *The Restoration of the Church of England, 1646–1689*, New Haven: Yale University Press.

____. (2003), 'A Sublime and Noble Service: John Evelyn and the Church of England', in *John Evelyn and his Milieu*, essays edited by Harris, Frances and Hunter, Michael, London: The British Library, pp. 145–63.

Stanley, Peter (2003), *For Fear of Pain: British Surgery, 1790–1850*, Amsterdam and New York: Rodopi.

Stearns, Peter N. and Stearns, Carol Z. (October 1985) 'Emotionology: Clarifying the History of Emotions and Emotional Standards', *American History Review*, **90**, pp. 813–36.

Stearns, Raymond Phineas (ed.) (1967), *A Journey to Paris In the Year 1698 by Martin Lister*, Bloomington: University of Illinois Press.

Stewart, Larry (1992), *The Rise of Public Science: Rhetoric, Technology and Natural Philosophy in Newtonian Britain, 1660–1750*, Cambridge: Cambridge University Press.

Stuart, Kathleen E. (1993), 'The Boundaries of Honor – Dishonorable people in Augsburg, 1500–1800', unpublished PhD thesis, New Haven, Conn.: Yale University.

Surtees Society (1882), *The Family Memoirs of the Rev. William Stukeley, M.D.*, London, **27** (73).

Thompson, Helen (2002), 'Plotting Materialism: W. Charleton's The Ephesian Matron, E. Haywood's Fantomina, and Feminine Consistency', *Eighteenth Century Studies*, **35** (2), pp. 185–214.

Thorpe, Clarence DeWitt (1940), *The Aesthetic Theory of Thomas Hobbes*, Ann Arbor: University of Michigan Press.

Todd, Margo (1983), 'Seneca and the Protestant Mind: The Influence of Stoicism on Puritan Ethics', *Archiv fur Reformationsgeschichte*, **74**, pp. 182–99.

Venn, John (1910), *The Works of John Caius, with a memoir of his life*, Cambridge: Cambridge University Press.

Villani, Stefano (2005), 'Between Anatomy and Politics: John Finch and Italy, 1649–1671', in Pelling, Margaret and Mandelbrote, Scott (eds), *The Practice of Reform in Health, Medicine, and Science, 1500–2000*, Aldershot and Burlington, Vt.: Ashgate Press, pp. 151–66.

Wade, Nicholas J. (2005), 'Medical Societies and Insanity in Late-Eighteenth Century London: The Fight between Andrew Marshal and John Hunter', *Journal of the History of the Neurosciences*, **14**, pp. 11–15.

Wear, Andrew (1985), 'Puritan perceptions of illness in Seventeenth-Century England', in Porter, Roy (ed.), *Patients and practitioners: Lay perceptions of medicine in pre-industrial society*, Cambridge and New York: Cambridge University Press, pp. 55–100.

____. (2000), *Knowledge and practice in English Medicine, 1550–1680*, Cambridge and New York: Cambridge University Press.

____. (1983), 'William Harvey and the "Way of the Anatomists"', *History of Science,* **21**, Pt. 3, (53), September, pp. 223–49.

____ (1985), 'Puritan perceptions of illness in Seventeenth-Century England', in Porter, Roy (ed.), *Patients and practitioners: Lay perceptions of medicine in pre-industrial society*, Cambridge and New York: Cambridge University Press, pp. 57–99.

Weatherall, D.J. (1994), 'The inhumanity of medicine', *British Medical Journal*, **309**, December 24–31, pp. 1671–2.

Webster, Charles (2002), *The Great Instauration, Science, Medicine and Reform, 1626–1660*, New York: Peter Lang.

____. (1967), 'The College of Physicians: "Solomon's House" in Commonwealth England', *Bulletin of the History of Medicine*, **41**, pp. 393–412.

____. (1977), 'Thomas Linacre and the foundation of the College of Physicians', in Maddison, Francis, Pelling, Margaret and Webster, Charles (eds), *Linacre Studies: Essays on the Life and Work of Thomas Linacre c. 1460–1524*, pp. 198–222, Oxford: Clarendon Press.

Whitteridge, Gweneth (1964), *The Anatomical Lectures of William Harvey*, Edinburgh: Livingstone Press.

____. (1971), *William Harvey and the Circulation of the Blood*, London: Macdonald.

____. (1971), *William Harvey and the Circulation of the Blood*, London: Macdonald.

Widess, J.D.H. (1980), *History of the Royal College of Ireland*, Edinburgh: Livingstone Press.

Williamson, George (1989), *Seventeenth Century Contexts*, Chicago: University of Chicago Press.

Wilson, Adrian (1995), *The Making of Man-Midwifery: Childbirth in England,1660–1770*, Cambridge, Mass.: Harvard University Press.

Wilson, Luke, (1987), 'William Harvey's *Prelectiones*: The Performance of the Body in the Renaissance Theater of Anatomy', *Representations*, **17**, Winter, pp. 62–95.

Wilson, Philip K. (1992), 'Acquiring surgical know-how: Occupational and lay instruction in early eighteenth-century London', in Porter, Roy (ed.), *The Popularisation of Medicine 1650–1850*, New York: Routledge Press, pp. 42–71.

____. (1992), 'Surgeon "turned" Physician: The Career and Writings of Daniel Turner 1667–1741', thesis, University College London.

____. (1999), *Surgery, Skin and Syphilis: Daniel Turner's London (1667–1741)*, Clio Medica, **54**, Amsterdam: Editions Rodolphi.

Wiltshire, John (1991), *Samuel Johnson in the Medical World: The Doctor and the Patient*, Cambridge: Cambridge University Press.

Winkler, Mary G. (Spring 1993), 'The Anatomical Theater', *Literature and Medicine,* **12**, (1), pp. 65–80.

Wright, John P. (1990), 'Hysteria and Mechanical Man', in Yolton, John W. (ed.), *Philosophy, Religion, and Science in the Seventeenth and Eighteenth Centuries*, Rochester: University of Rochester Press, pp. 233–47.

Young, Sidney (ed.) (1890), *Annals of the Barber Surgeons of London*, London.

Index

(References to illustrations are in **bold**)